South Beach Diet

Best Collection of South Beach Diet Recipes Full of Healthy Fats

Kickstart Meal Plan for Living and Eating Well Every Day

2 BOOKS in 1

Emma Green

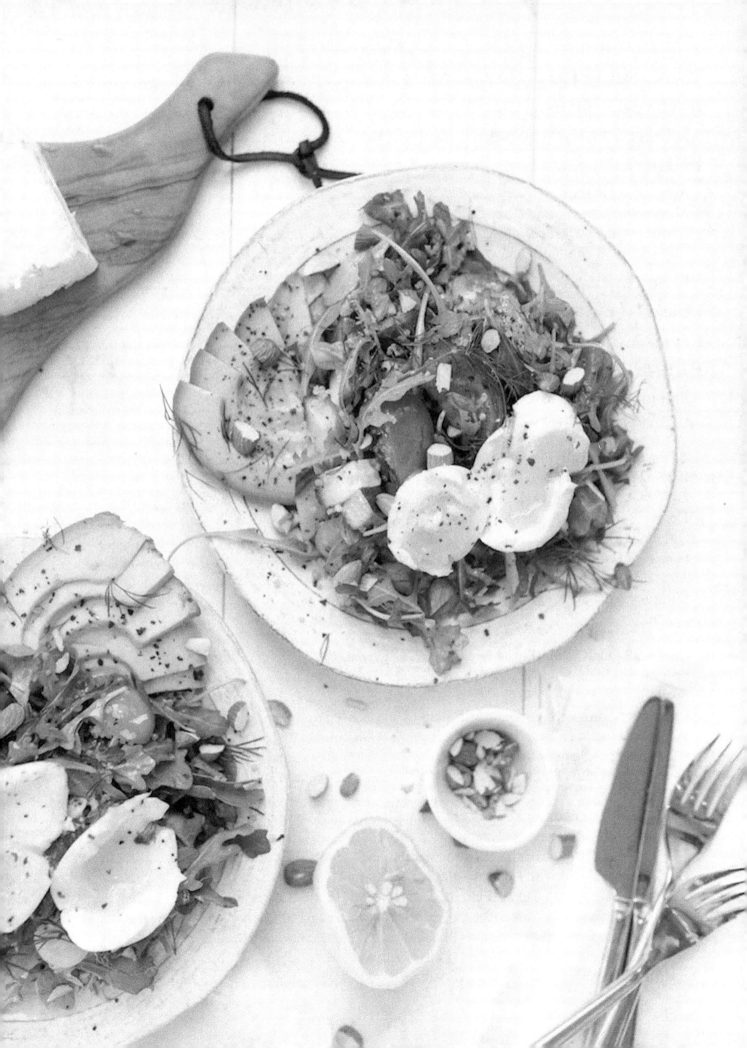

CONTENTS

South Beach Diet

Beginner's Guide with Foolproof Recipes

Lose Weight Easily and Reduce Your Risk of Heart Disease

Emma Green

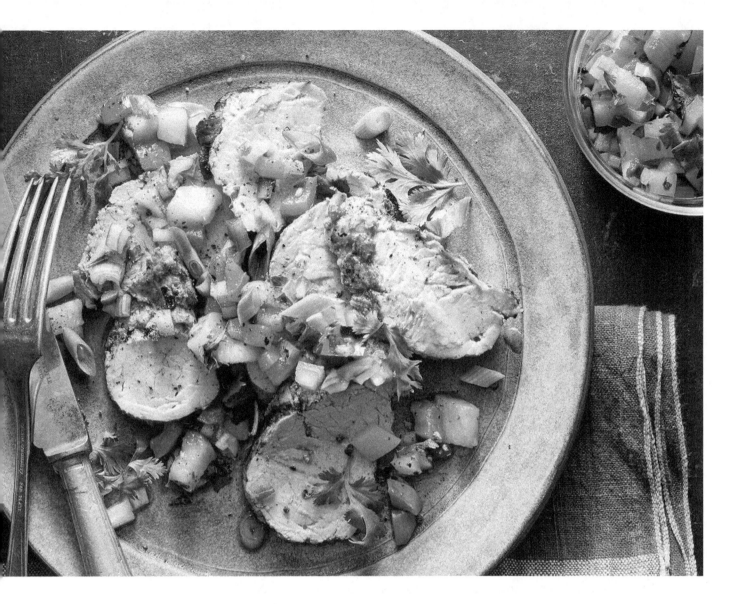

INTRODUCTION

For everyone who has struggled with weight loss and related health issues in the past, there is great news: The diet debates are over! After decades of confusing messages—"low fat" one day, "low carb" the next day, and "cabbage soup" the day after that— a consensus regarding the principles of healthy eating has been achieved. Experts agree that we should be consuming the "right fats," the "right carbohydrates," "lean sources of Protein –," and "plenty of fiber." These are the principles of the South Beach Diet, and they have been successfully used for weight loss and better health by millions of people around the world. The South Beach Diet is intended to be more than just a diet. It is a good stimulus to overcome the poor eating habits and sedentary lifestyle that are making us fatter and sicker every day.

This cookbook offers many easy and delicious recipes that you can enjoy while you lose weight and improve your overall health. As you eat better, you'll not only look and feel better but also improve your blood chemistry and reduce your risk for diabetes and a host of other diseases.

The book also includes many recipes that take less than 15 minutes to prepare, plus quick-cook ideas. In the same amount of time that it takes to pick up an order at a fast-food restaurant, you'll be able to prepare delicious, healthy meals. You'll see that it is possible to have a "fast-food" lifestyle that is also nutritious. In fact, the meals in this cookbook are so flavorful that your family may not even realize that they are also good for them!

A Closer Look at the South Beach Diet

All the food we consume contains a large and wide number of nutrients. These can be divided *into* si
general *categories*: water, Protein –s, carbohydrates (carbs), fats, *vitamins*, and minerals. The carbs and
the fats can be both good and bad. Success in losing weight is found by preferring the best of each. Tha
means lots of vegetables, fish, eggs, dairy, lean Protein – like chicken and turkey, whole grains, and nuts
The South Beach Diet is not high in carbohydrates but high in Protein – and healthy fats.

The diet doesn't banish all carbs. The ones you do consume are low on the glycemic index (GI), a
estimate of how carbs affect blood glucose.

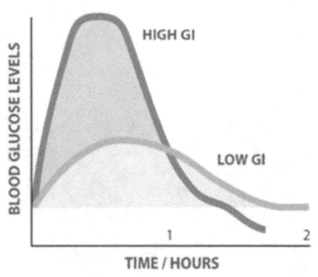

The amount of carbohydrate in the reference
and test food must be the same.

Low-GI "good" carbs are known to keep your blood sugar and metabolism at healthy levels, and to keep
you feeling fuller longer, while high-GI "bad" carbs have the opposite effect.

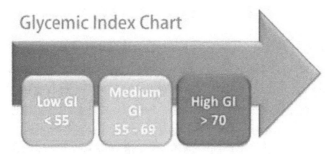

This book concentrates mostly on Phase I recipes as this phase is the most carb restrictive one. Practically
any Phase I recipe can also be a Phase II recipe simply by serving it with additional carbs. For example
you can eat guacamole with celery stalks on Phase I or add buttered toast for Phase II. You can add 1-
diced carrots to any of your soups and it becomes Phase II friendly.

Phase I

The first phase of the South Beach Diet is two weeks long and rich in lean Protein –, low-fat dairy and high-fiber vegetables. During this phase you will be enjoying three normal well-balanced meals a day with snacks in between. At the same time this is the most carb restrictive phase and it eliminates cravings. The foods you will not be enjoying throughout the first phase are the following:

- **Fruit**: All kinds of fruits including dried fruit and fruit juices are to be avoided in this stage.
- **Vegetables**: Carrots, beets, potatoes, green peas, corn, turnip, or other starchy vegetables are to cut out.
- **Starches:** Bread, pastries, pasta, rice, cereal, oatmeal, matzo are out of the question.
- **Meat and poultry:** Fatty cuts like brisket or rib steaks, dark meat poultry products, duck, and ham are also to be avoided.
- **Dairy:** no whole or 2% milk.
- **All alcohol beverages** are restricted.
- **Sweets**: Candies and treats containing sugar as well as ice cream are eliminated.

Allowed vegetables chart

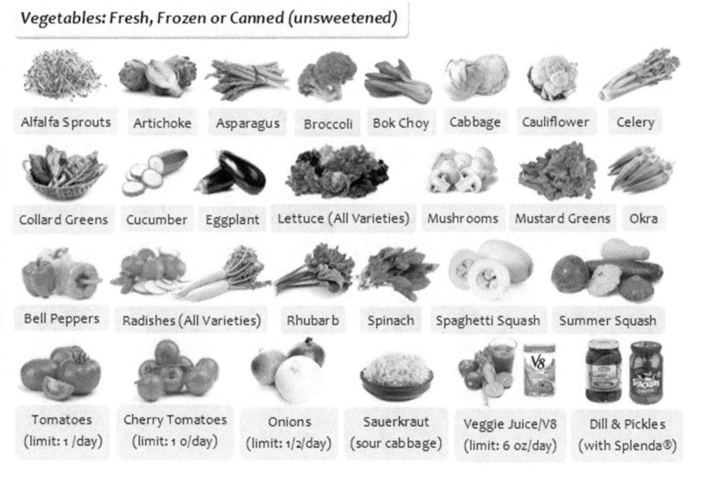

Vegetables: Fresh, Frozen or Canned (unsweetened)

Alfalfa Sprouts · Artichoke · Asparagus · Broccoli · Bok Choy · Cabbage · Cauliflower · Celery

Collard Greens · Cucumber · Eggplant · Lettuce (All Varieties) · Mushrooms · Mustard Greens · Okra

Bell Peppers · Radishes (All Varieties) · Rhubarb · Spinach · Spaghetti Squash · Summer Squash

Tomatoes (limit: 1 /day) · Cherry Tomatoes (limit: 1 o/day) · Onions (limit: 1/2/day) · Sauerkraut (sour cabbage) · Veggie Juice/V8 (limit: 6 oz/day) · Dill & Pickles (with Splenda®)

Allowed legumes

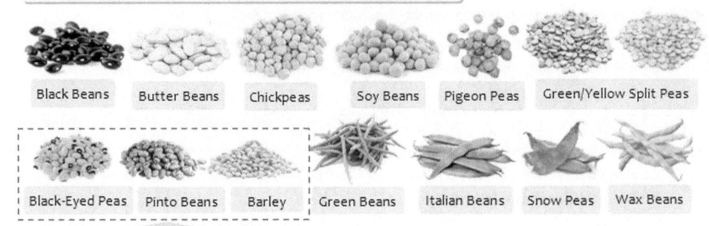

Beans & Legumes: Fresh, Frozen or Canned (unsweetened)

Black Beans · Butter Beans · Chickpeas · Soy Beans · Pigeon Peas · Green/Yellow Split Peas

Black-Eyed Peas · Pinto Beans · Barley · Green Beans · Italian Beans · Snow Peas · Wax Beans

ONLY ALLOWED IN PHASE 2

Allowed sauces and seasonings

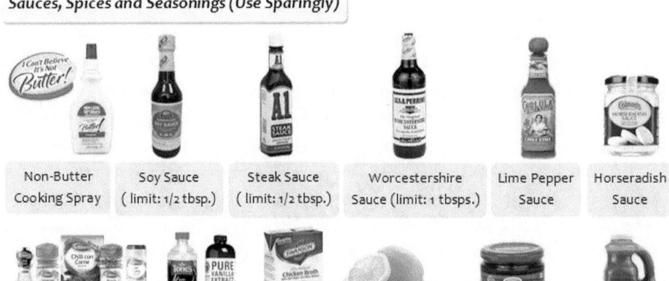

Sauces, Spices and Seasonings (Use Sparingly)

Non-Butter Cooking Spray · Soy Sauce (limit: 1/2 tbsp.) · Steak Sauce (limit: 1/2 tbsp.) · Worcestershire Sauce (limit: 1 tbsps.) · Lime Pepper Sauce · Horseradish Sauce

All Spices (no added sugar) · Extracts (Almond, etc.) · Broth (Fat-free) · Fresh Lemon Juice · Salsa Dip (Phase 1 limit: 2 tbsps.) · Hot Sauce

Allowed meat chart

Beef: Lean cuts

Top Round   Eye of Round   Tenderloin   Top Loin

Ground Beef
(extra lean 96/4, lean 92/8, sirloin 90/10)

Lamb: All visible fat removed

Loin   Center Cut   Loin Chop

Lunchmeat: Fat-free or Low-fat

Pork

Loin   Tenderloin   Canadian Bacon

Boiled Ham

Veal

Top Round   Chop   Leg Cutlets

Meat Products: <3gms fat per 3-oz portion

Bacon   Burger   Sausage Patties

Hotdog

Seafood: All fish & Shellfish

Bacon: Limit to 2 slices per day

Sausage Pattie : Limit to 1 patty per day

Phase II

The aim of the second phase of the South Beach Diet is to define your personally correct carb level and reach your personal target weight. The phase is strictly individual and may be of different lengths for different people. It may be broken into six weeks during which you gradually restore your carbs:

Week 1. The plan of the first week of Phase II is to eat one serving of a carbohydrate food each day experimenting to see how you feel. This will be a serving of fresh fruit for either breakfast or lunch or dinner.

Week 2. This week you will be enjoying each day one serving of fresh fruit plus one serving of high-fiber starchy foods, e.g. beans or other legumes.

Week 3. This week again another serving per day of carbs will be added and bread can be an option. It is better to choose bread with more fiber and less starch.

Week 4. Add another serving of carbohydrate food.

Week 5. Add one more serving of carbs.

Week 6. Add another serving of cards and by this time you will be having three servings of fruit and three servings of grains or starches each day.

Going through the second phase implies slow weight loss and will last as long as it takes you to lose your desired weight.

Phase III

Phase III of the South Beach diet is meant for weight maintenance. No food is off limits here as long as you maintain your correct weight. You are still encouraged to eat "good" carbs, such as whole-grain bread, brown rice, whole-wheat pasta and fruit, but they are already in your lifestyle once you get to this phase. Your diet has definitely become greener, however you can enjoy indulging in a special, decadent treat on occasion. Live every day to the fullest— in moderation.

Pros & Cons

Pros:

- Enhances heart health
- Boosts weight loss
- Reduces hunger
- Stabilizes blood sugar level

Cons:

- Forbids some healthy, beneficial fats
- Encourages Omega 6 vegetable oils
- Permits artificial sweeteners

BREAKFAST
Buttermilk Waffles with Jam
(Phase II)

Prep time: 10 minutes

Cooking time: 20 minutes

Servings: 4

Nutrients per serving:

Carbohydrates – 56 g

Fat – 15 g

Protein – 11 g

Calories – 360

Ingredients:

- 1 cup whole-wheat flour
- 1 cup old-fashioned rolled oats
- 1 Tbsp plus 1 tsp baking powder
- Salt to taste
- 3 Tbsp granular sugar substitute
- 3 Tbsp canola oil
- 1¼ cups 1 percent or fat-free buttermilk
- ½ cup water
- 1 large egg
- ¾ cup sugar-free jam, any flavor

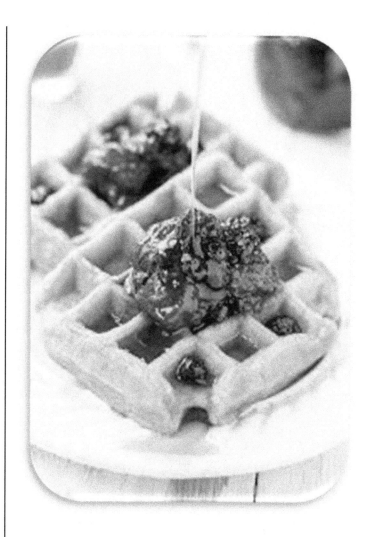

Instructions:

1. In a bowl, mix together the first five ingredients.
2. In another bowl, whisk together the oil, buttermilk, water, and egg. Combine the two mixtures and mix well.
3. Heat waffle iron; coat with cooking spray. Add ½ cup batter per waffle and cook until browned and crisp, about 5 minutes. Dollop with jam and serve.

Greet-the-Sun Breakfast Pizzas
(Phase II)

Prep time: 10 minutes

Cooking time: 8 minutes

Servings: 2

Nutrients per serving:

Carbohydrates – 56 g

Fat – 15 g

Protein – 11 g

Calories – 360

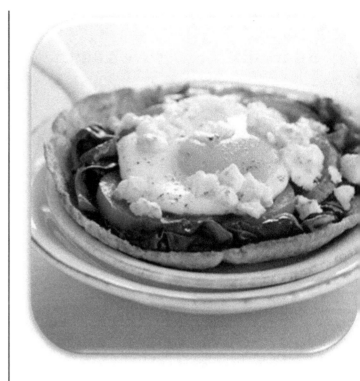

Ingredients:

- 5 tsp extra-virgin olive oil
- 1 onion, chopped
- 1 bell pepper,chopped
- 1½ tsp Italian seasoning
- 4 ounces packed spinach (4 cups)
- 2 (6-inch) whole-grain pitas, halved horizontally
- 2 large plum tomatoes, thinly sliced
- 4 large eggs
- ¼ tsp salt
- ¼ tsp black pepper
- 2 ounces reduced-fat feta cheese, crumbled

Instructions:

1. Heat 1 tsp of the oil in a nonstick skillet. Add onion and cook for 3 minutes. Add bell pepper, tomato, and Italian seasoning; cook for another 3 minutes.
2. Heat the oven to 350°F.
3. Divide spinach and the cooked vegetables equally among pita halves, leaving an empty space in the center for an egg.
4. Crack 1 egg into the center of each. Sprinkle with cheese, salt, and pepper, and place petas on a baking sheet. Transfer to the oven, and bake until yolks are lightly set, 8 to 10 minutes. Serve.

Wholesome Oat Muffins (Phase II)

Prep time: 10 minutes

Cooking time: 15 minutes

Servings: 12

Nutrients per serving:

Carbohydrates – 18 g

Fat – 11 g

Protein – 4 g

Calories – 179

Ingredients:

- 1 cup buttermilk
- ¾ cup plus 2 Tbsp rolled oats
- 1¼ cups whole-grain pastry flour
- 1½ tsp baking powder
- ½ tsp baking soda
- ¼ tsp ground cinnamon
- ¼ tsp salt
- ⅔ cup chopped walnuts
- ⅓ cup granular brown sugar substitute
- ⅓ cup canola oil
- 1 large egg, beaten
- 1 tsp vanilla extract

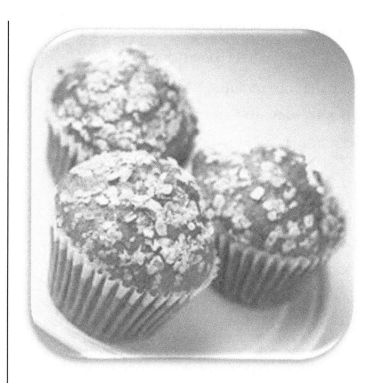

Instructions:

1. Preheat the oven to 425°F. Coat a 12-cup nonstick muffin pan with cooking spray.
2. In a small bowl, combine buttermilk and ¾ cup of the oats. Let soak for 30 minutes.
3. In another bowl, mix flour, baking powder, baking soda, cinnamon, and salt. Stir in walnuts.
4. In a large bowl, mix brown sugar substitute, oil, egg, and vanilla until well blended. Stir in the oats mixture and the flour mixture until just combined.
5. Divide batter among the muffin cups (about two-thirds full). Sprinkle remaining 2 Tbsp oats over muffins. Bake for about 15 minutes.
6. Let cool for 5 minutes. Remove muffins to a rack to cool.

Three Berry–Stuffed French Toast (Phase II)

Prep time: 10 minutes

Cooking time: 10 minutes

Servings: 4

Nutrients per serving:

Carbohydrates – 30 g

Fat – 9 g

Protein – 17 g

Calories – 280

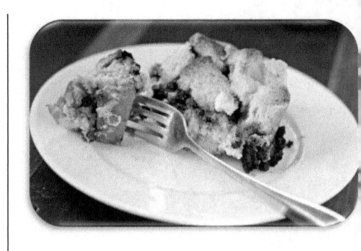

Ingredients:

- ⅓ cup blackberries
- ⅓ cup blueberries
- ⅓ cup raspberries
- ⅔ cup semisoft farmer's cheese
- 1 Tbsp granular sugar substitute
- 8 slices whole-grain sandwich bread
- 3 large eggs
- ¼ cup 1% milk
- ¼ tsp ground cinnamon

Instructions:

1. In a bowl, combine first five ingredients. Mash them together with a fork. Spread the berry mixture on 4 slices of the bread and top with the remaining bread slices to form 4 sandwiches.

2. In a shallow dish, beat eggs, milk, and cinnamon. Dip sandwiches into egg mixture to coat both sides.

3. Coat a nonstick skillet with cooking spray and heat over medium heat. Cook French toast in two batches for about 2 minutes per side. Serve warm.

Blackberry-Banana Breakfast Smoothies (Phase II)

Prep time: 10 minutes

Cooking time: none

Servings: 4

Nutrients per serving:

Carbohydrates – 21 g

Fat – 0.5 g

Protein – 5 g

Calories – 100

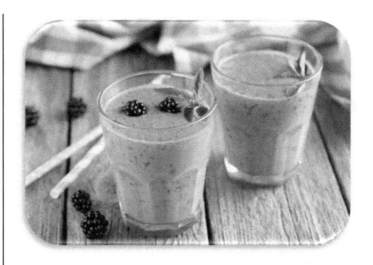

Ingredients:

- 2 small bananas, quartered
- 1 cup blackberries, plus extra for garnish
- 1½ cups low-fat plain yogurt
- 1 Tbsp granular sugar substitute
- 1 Tbsp wheat germ
- 4 ice cubes

Instructions:

1. In a blender, combine bananas and blackberries; purée until smooth. Add remaining ingredients; blend for about 1 minute. Pour into 4 (10-ounce) glasses, garnish with whole blackberries and serve.

Orange-Blueberry Breakfast Muffins (Phase II)

Prep time: 15 minutes

Cooking time: 35 minutes

Servings: 12

Nutrients per serving:

Carbohydrates – 20 g

Fat – 5 g

Protein – 4 g

Calories – 132

Ingredients:

- ¾ cup quinoa flakes, toasted
- 1 cup sorghum flour
- 2 Tbsp chia seeds, finely ground
- 2 Tbsp granulated stevia (baking formula)
- 2 tsp gluten-free baking powder
- ½ tsp baking soda
- ½ tsp xanthan gum
- ¼ tsp salt
- 1 cup light (1.5%) buttermilk
- 3 Tbsp extra-virgin olive oil
- ⅓ cup liquid egg whites (or the whites of 2 large eggs)
- 2 Tbsp agave nectar
- 2 tsp grated orange zest
- 1¼ cups fresh or frozen blueberries (no need to thaw)

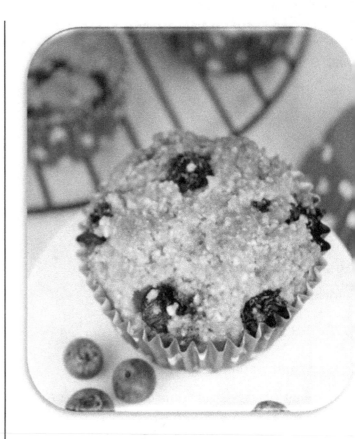

Instructions:

1. Preheat the oven to 375°F. Line a standard 12-cup muffin pan with paper liners. Place the quinoa flakes on a baking sheet and toast until fragrant and crisp, about 15 minutes.
2. In a large bowl, stir together the sorghum flour, chia seeds, stevia, baking powder, baking soda, xanthan gum, and salt.
3. In a medium bowl, whisk together the buttermilk, oil, egg whites, agave nectar, and orange zest. Make a well in the center of the dry ingredients, pour in the buttermilk mixture, and stir gently to combine. Fold in the blueberries.
4. Divide the batter among the muffin cups.
5. Bake for 17 to 20 minutes. Let cool before serving.

Hearty Buttermilk Pancakes with Sautéed Apples (Phase II)

Prep time: 15 minutes

Cooking time: 10 minutes

Servings: 4

Nutrients per serving:

Carbohydrates – 39 g

Fat – 8.5 g

Protein – 11 g

Calories – 268

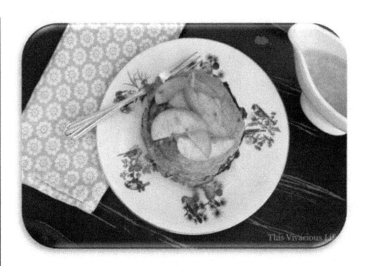

Ingredients:

- 2 large apples, peeled (about 8 ounces each), cored, halved, and thinly sliced
- 1 Tbsp fresh lemon juice
- ½ cup chickpea flour
- ½ cup 100% buckwheat flour
- 2 Tbsp cornmeal
- 1½ tsp gluten-free baking powder
- ½ tsp baking soda
- ⅛ tsp salt
- 1¼ cups light (1.5%) buttermilk
- 1 large egg
- ⅓ cup liquid egg whites (or the whites of 2 large eggs)
- 1 Tbsp plus 1 tsp extra-virgin olive oil

Instructions:

1. In a large skillet, toss the apple slices with the lemon juice and 3 Tbsp water and cook over medium heat for about 3 minutes. Remove from the heat and cover to keep warm while you make the pancakes.

2. In a bowl, mix together the chickpea flour, buckwheat flour, cornmeal, baking powder, baking soda, and salt.

3. In a separate large bowl or large glass measuring cup, combine the buttermilk, whole egg, egg whites, and oil. Stir the liquid ingredients into the dry ingredients until no lumps remain.

4. Coat a large nonstick skillet with olive oil cooking spray. Heat the skillet over medium-low heat and ladle a scant ¼ cup batter per pancake into the pan. Cook for about 2 minutes, then flip them over and cook until the undersides are done, about 1 minute. Repeat with the remaining batter.

5. Serve the pancakes topped with the apple slices and any juice.

Quiche Lorraine Minis (Phase II)

Prep time: 15 minutes

Cooking time: 45 minutes

Servings: 4

Nutrients per serving:

Carbohydrates – 15 g

Fat – 8 g

Protein – 19 g

Calories – 213

Ingredients:

- olive oil cooking spray
- 1 tsp extra-virgin olive oil
- 4 ounces gluten-free Canadian bacon, coarsely chopped
- ¾ cup chickpea flour
- 1 can (12 ounces) fat-free evaporated milk
- 6 Tbsp liquid egg whites
- 1 whole egg
- 2 tsp Dijon mustard
- Freshly ground black pepper, ground nutmeg, to taste
- 1 cup shredded reduced-fat Swiss cheese (4 ounces)

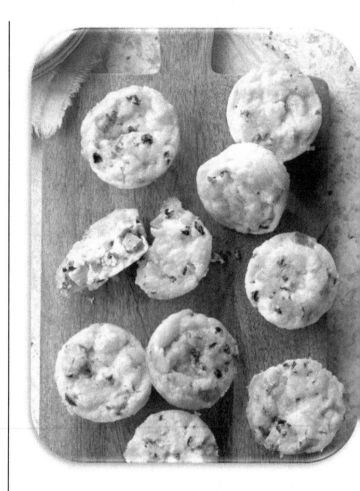

Instructions:

1. Preheat the oven to 350°F. Use a jumbo muffin pan and if it isn't nonstick, lightly coat the cups with olive oil cooking spray.
2. In a nonstick skillet, heat the oil. Add the Canadian bacon and cook, stirring often, until lightly browned, 4 to 5 minutes.
3. In a bowl, whisk the chickpea flour, evaporated milk, egg whites, whole egg, mustard, pepper, and nutmeg until just blended.
4. Divide the bacon among the muffin cups. Divide the cheese among the cups. Pour the custard mixture over the cheese and bacon (the cups will be about three-fourths full).
5. Bake until nicely browned on top and cooked through but still moist, 30 to 35 minutes. Transfer to a rack to cool slightly. Serve warm or at room temperature.

Sausage and Scrambled Egg Breakfast Tostadas (Phase II)

Prep time: 20 minutes

Cooking time: 25 minutes

Servings: 4

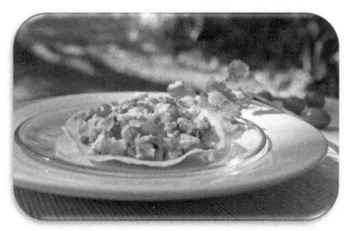

Nutrients per serving:

Carbohydrates – 15 g

Fat – 8 g

Protein – 20 g

Calories – 243

Ingredients:

- ¼ cup chopped grape tomatoes
- 2 scallions, thinly sliced
- Coarse kosher salt
- Gluten-free chili powder
- 4 (6-inch) 100% corn tortillas
- Olive oil cooking spray
- 2 Italian-style turkey sausage links
- 1 Tbsp extra-virgin olive oil
- 1 green bell pepper, finely diced
- 1 small onion, finely diced
- 2 large eggs
- ½ cup liquid egg whites
- ¼ cup shredded reduced-fat Mexican-blend cheese
- ¼ cup nonfat (0%) plain Greek yogurt

Instructions:

1. In a bowl, toss together the tomatoes, scallions, and a small pinch each of salt and chili powder. Set this fresh salsa aside.

2. Preheat the broiler. Put the tortillas on a baking sheet and coat with olive oil cooking spray. Sprinkle each with a pinch of chili powder. Broil for 2 to 3 minutes. Set the tortillas aside.

3. In a large skillet, bring a ½ inch of water to a boil. Pierce the sausages in several places, add to the skillet, cover, and cook, turning once, for about 7 minutes. Dice them when cool enough to handle.

4. Wipe out the skillet, add the oil and heat over medium-high heat. Add the bell pepper and onion and cook for about 7 minutes.

5. In another bowl, beat together the whole eggs and egg whites. Add the egg mixture and diced sausage to the skillet and scramble to your preferred doneness. Sprinkle the cheese over the eggs and let sit a minute to melt.

6. Top each tortilla with eggs (a generous ½ cup each) and a tablespoon each of the yogurt and salsa.

Almond-Pear Quinoa Breakfast Cereal (Phase II)

Prep time: 15 minutes

Cooking time: 20 minutes

Servings: 4

Nutrients per serving:

Carbohydrates – 45 g

Fat – 5.5 g

Protein – 11 g

Calories – 269

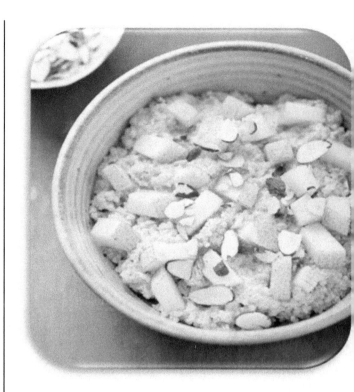

Ingredients:

- 1¼ cups quinoa, rinsed
- ¼ tsp fine sea salt
- 1 cup unsweetened almond milk
- ¼ tsp ground cinnamon
- 1 juicy ripe pear
- ½ tsp pure vanilla extract
- 1 cup fat-free milk, unsweetened almond milk, or unsweetened low-fat soy
- milk
- 2 Tbsp sliced almonds (toasted, if desired)
- Monk fruit natural no-calorie sweetener, for serving (optional)

Instructions:

1. In a medium nonstick saucepan, combine the quinoa, salt, and 1 cup water. Bring to a boil, reduce to a high simmer, cover, and cook until partially cooked about 6 minutes.

2. Meanwhile, place the almond milk (or another choice) and cinnamon in a small bowl. Core the pear and grate it on the large holes of a box grater, and add it to the almond milk. Stir to submerge the pear gratings.

3. Uncover the saucepan and add the almond milk mixture. Return to a simmer, cover, and cook, stirring occasionally, until the quinoa is tender and the milk is mostly absorbed 9 to 11 minutes.

4. Remove the pan from the heat and add the vanilla. Serve with ¼ cup milk per serving and topped with the almonds (1½ tsp per serving) and a sprinkling of monk fruit sweetener, if desired.

Summer Squash Scramble with Fresh Tomato (Phase I)

Prep time: 15 minutes

Cooking time: 10 minutes

Servings: 2

Nutrients per serving:

Carbohydrates – 8 g

Fat – 12 g

Protein – 11 g

Calories – 180

Ingredients:

- 3 large eggs
- 1 tsp chopped chives
- Salt, pepper to taste
- 2 tsp canola oil
- 1 yellow summer squash, halved and thinly sliced into half-moons
- ½ small onion, chopped
- 1 medium tomato, chopped

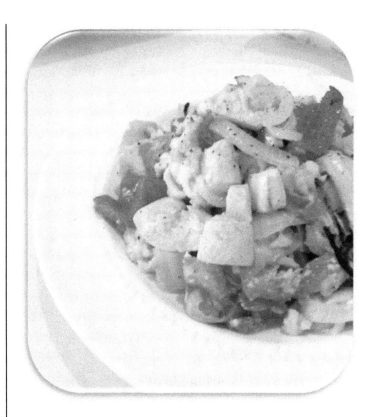

Instructions:

1. In a bowl, beat together eggs, chives, salt, and pepper.
2. In a nonstick skillet, heat oil over medium heat. Cook squash and onion, stirring occasionally, for about 8 minutes.
3. Add the egg mixture to the skillet and cook, stirring frequently, for about 2 minutes.
4. Serve eggs warm on 2 plates, topped with tomato.

LUNCH

Curried Squash Soup (Phase I)

Prep time: 15 minutes

Cooking time: 15 minutes

Servings: 4

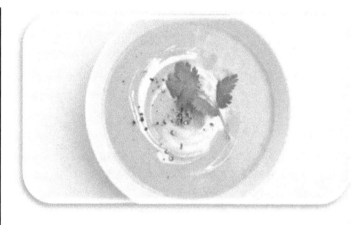

Nutrients per serving:

Carbohydrates – 30 g

Fat – 5 g

Protein – 10 g

Calories – 200

Ingredients:

- 1 Tbsp extra-virgin olive oil
- 2 tsp curry powder
- 2 medium yellow squash, chopped (3 cups)
- 1 large onion, coarsely chopped
- 3 cups low-sodium chicken broth
- 1 (15.5-ounce) can chickpeas, rinsed and drained
- Freshly ground black pepper
- Salt to taste
- ½ cup nonfat plain yogurt
- 2 Tbsp fresh basil, chopped

Instructions:

1. In a large saucepan, heat oil over medium-high heat. Add curry powder and chickpeas, bring to a simmer, and remove from the heat.
2. Transfer 2 cups of the soup to a blender and purée until smooth. Return puréed soup to the pan with the rest of the soup and stir to combine. Season with salt and pepper to taste.
3. Refrigerate until chilled, about 45 minutes.
4. Divide soup among 4 bowls, top with a dollop of yogurt and a sprinkling of basil, and serve.

Summery Melon Soup (Phase II)

Prep time: 20 minutes

Cooking time: none

Servings: 4

Nutrients per serving:

Carbohydrates – 24 g

Fat – 1 g

Protein – 3 g

Calories – 110

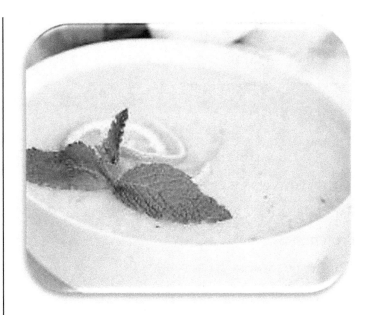

Ingredients:

- ½ (5-pound) honeydew peeled and chopped (5 cups)
- 1 large cucumber, peeled and chopped
- ½ cup low-fat plain yogurt
- 2 scallions, roughly chopped
- 1 Tbsp fresh lemon juice
- 2 tsp finely grated lemon zest

Instructions:

1. In a blender, purée honeydew until smooth. Add cucumber, yogurt, scallions, lemon juice, and 1 tsp of the zest; purée until smooth. Refrigerate until chilled, about 30 minutes.
2. Sprinkle with 1 tsp zest before serving.

Sweet Potato Vichyssoise (Phase II)

Prep time: 15 minutes

Cooking time: 20 minutes

Servings: 4

Nutrients per serving:

Carbohydrates – 24 g

Fat – 4 g

Protein – 7 g

Calories – 160

Ingredients:

- medium sweet potatoes (1 ½pounds), peeled, cut into 1-inch chunks
- 1 Tbsp extra-virgin olive oil
- medium leeks, roots, and tops trimmed and discarded, whites chopped (3 cups)
- 1 cup low-sodium chicken broth
- cups fat-free milk
- ¼ tsp salt
- 1 Tbsp chopped chives

Instructions:

1. Place sweet potatoes in a saucepan and add water to cover. Bring to a low boil and cook until sweet potatoes have softened about 15 minutes. Drain in a colander and let cool briefly.

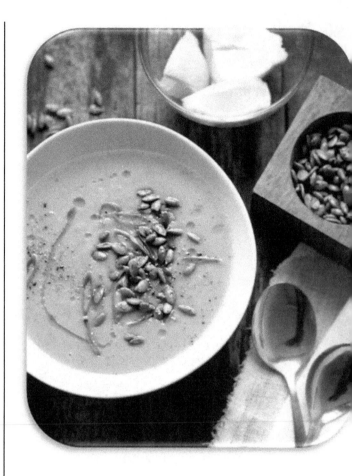

2. While sweet potatoes are cooking, heat the oil over medium heat in a medium nonstick skillet . Add leeks, cover, and cook for about 5 minutes. Add broth, bring to a simmer, and cook for 3 minute more. Remove from the heat and let cool.

3. In a blender, combine sweet potatoes, leeks, and broth; purée for 1 minute. Add milk and salt; purée until smooth. Refrigerate for about 45 minutes.

4. Divide soup among 4 bowls, sprinkle with chives and serve.

Cucumber Soup with Grilled Shrimp and Dill (Phase I)

Prep time: 20 minutes

Cooking time: 5 minutes

Servings: 4

Nutrients per serving:

Carbohydrates – 24 g

Fat – 2.5 g

Protein – 19 g

Calories – 140

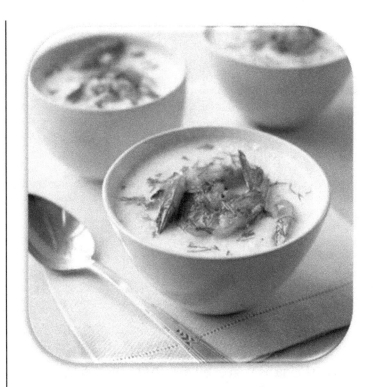

Ingredients:

- 2 large cucumbers, peeled, seeded and roughly chopped
- ¾ cup cold water
- 1 cup low-fat or nonfat plain yogurt
- 1 Tbsp fresh lime juice
- ¼ tsp salt
- ¼ tsp freshly ground black pepper
- ¾ pound large shrimp, heads removed, peeled, deveined
- ¼ cup chopped fresh dill

Instructions:

1. In a blender, combine cucumbers and water; purée for 30 seconds. Add yogurt, lime juice, salt, and pepper; purée until smooth.
2. Coat a grill with cooking spray. Grill shrimp on medium heat for about 1 minute per side.
3. Divide soup among 4 bowls, top with shrimp and dill, and serve.

White Gazpacho (Phase II)

Prep time: 20 minutes

Cooking time: none

Servings: 4

Nutrients per serving:

Carbohydrates – 14 g

Fat – 9 g

Protein – 6 g

Calories – 150

Ingredients:

- 1 slice whole-grain bread, crust removed
- 1½ cups vegetable broth
- ½ cup slivered almonds
- 1 large cucumber, peeled and chopped
- 1 medium yellow bell pepper, chopped
- 4 scallions, chopped
- 1 Tbsp red wine vinegar
- 6 seedless green grapes, halved

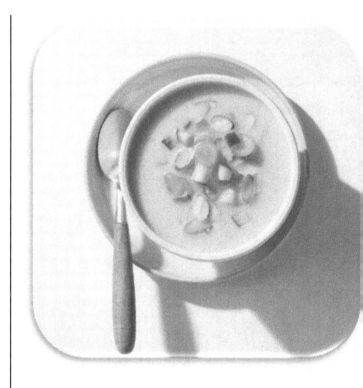

Instructions:

1. Place bread in a blender and cover with broth; let sit until bread begins to soften, about 3 minutes.
2. Reserve 2 Tbsp of the almonds; add remaining 6 Tbsp almonds to the blender with the broth and purée until very smooth, about 1 minute. Add cucumber, pepper, scallions, and vinegar to the blender; purée until mixture is slightly chunky.
3. Refrigerate soup in a covered container for about 30 minutes. To serve, divide soup among 4 bowls and top with reserved almonds and grape halves.

Garden White Bean Soup (Phase I)

Prep time: 25 minutes

Cooking time: 25 minutes

Servings: 4

Nutrients per serving:

Carbohydrates – 40 g

Fat – 8 g

Protein – 17 g

Calories – 290

Ingredients:

- 1 Tbsp plus 2 tsp extra-virgin olive oil
- 1 medium onion, thinly sliced
- 4 garlic cloves, thinly sliced
- 1 celery stalk, thinly sliced
- Pinch red pepper flakes
- 2 (15-ounce) cans cannellini beans, rinsed and drained
- 3 cups low-sodium chicken broth
- 1½ cups packed chopped arugula
- ¼ cup packed basil leaves, chopped
- ¼ tsp grated lemon zest
- ¼ tsp salt
- 4 Tbsp freshly grated Parmesan cheese

Instructions:

1. In a saucepan, heat 1 Tbsp of the oil over medium heat. Add onion, garlic, celery, and pepper flakes. Cook on low until

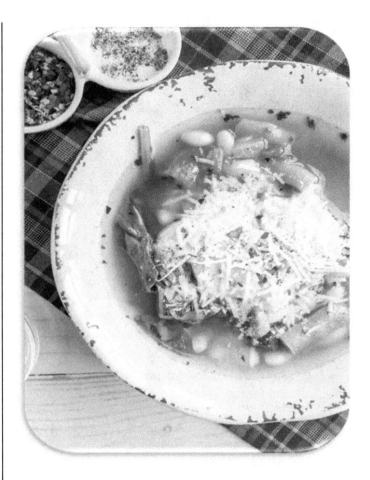

vegetables are softened, 10 to 12 minutes. Add beans and broth, bring to a simmer, and cook for 10 minutes. Remove from the heat and carefully strain liquid into a large bowl.

2. Transfer bean mixture in the strainer to a blender or food processor, add 1 cup of the reserved liquid, remaining 2 tsp oil, arugula, basil, lemon zest, and salt; purée until smooth. Add to the bowl with the rest of the reserved cooking liquid and stir to combine.

3. Serve warm in 4 bowls, sprinkled with cheese.

Savory Egg Salad (Phase II)

Prep time: 15 minutes

Cooking time: 10 minutes

Servings: 4

Nutrients per serving:

Carbohydrates – 2 g

Fat – 15 g

Protein – 11 g

Calories – 190

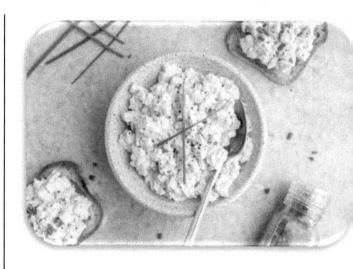

Ingredients:

- 8 large eggs
- ½ small red onion, minced
- 2 celery stalks, minced
- 4 large green olives, chopped (optional)
- 3 Tbsp mayonnaise
- 1 tsp Dijon mustard
- ¼ tsp salt
- 1½ cups baby arugula

Instructions:

1. In a saucepan, bring eggs to a boil. Remove from the heat, cover, and let eggs sit for 20 minutes. Peel eggs when cool enough.
2. In a medium bowl, mash 5 whole boiled eggs and 3 boiled egg whites together with the back of a fork. Add the remaining ingredients; stir to combine. Serve.

Grilled Salmon Salad (Phase II)

Prep time: 15 minutes

Cooking time: 12 minutes

Servings: 4

Nutrients per serving:

Carbohydrates – 19 g

Fat – 14 g

Protein – 28 g

Calories – 310

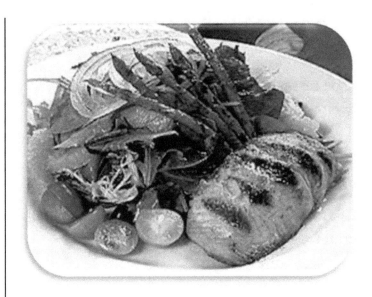

Ingredients:

- 1 pound skinless salmon fillet, about 1 inch thick
- 1½ cups watercress leaves, chopped
- 1 medium cucumber, peeled, seeded and chopped
- 2 Tbsp reduced-fat sour cream
- 1 Tbsp fresh lemon juice
- 1 Tbsp chopped fresh dill
- 8 slices thin-sliced whole-wheat bread

Instructions:

1. Coat a grill with cooking spray. Grill salmon until opaque in the center, 4 to 5 minutes per side. Let cool.
2. In a bowl, combine watercress, cucumber, sour cream, lemon juice, and dill. Flake cooled salmon into the bowl; toss well.
3. serve.Transfer to the serving plates. Serve.

Bounty Greek Salad (Phase I)

Prep time: 15 minutes

Cooking time: 15 minutes

Servings: 4

Nutrients per serving:

Carbohydrates – 13 g

Fat – 3 g

Protein – 9 g

Calories – 180

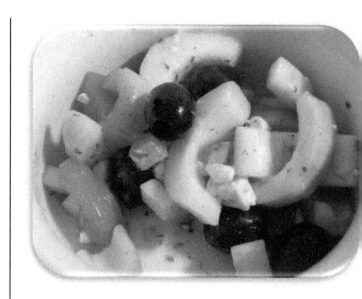

Ingredients:

- 8 ounces green beans, trimmed
- 1 (12-ounce) head romaine lettuce, chopped (6 cups)
- 2 medium tomatoes, cut into wedges
- 1 medium cucumber, halved lengthwise, seeded, and thinly sliced
- 4 ounces reduced-fat feta cheese, crumbled
- ¼ cup pitted kalamata olives, sliced
- 2 Tbsp extra-virgin olive oil
- 1 Tbsp red wine vinegar
- ⅛ tsp salt
- ⅛ tsp freshly ground black pepper
- ¼ cup chopped fresh parsley

Instructions:

1. In a saucepan, bring salted water to a boil. Add beans and cook for about 3 minutes. Drain in a colander. Pat dry. Cut beans into 1-inch pieces.
2. In a large bowl, combine beans, lettuce, tomatoes, cucumber, feta, and olives. In a bowl, whisk together oil, vinegar, salt, and pepper; pour over salad and toss to coat. Divide salad among 4 plates and sprinkle with parsley just before serving.

Endive Salad with Walnuts (Phase I)

Prep time: 10 minutes

Cooking time: 10 minutes

Servings: 4

Nutrients per serving:

Carbohydrates – 6 g

Fat – 12 g

Protein – 3 g

Calories – 130

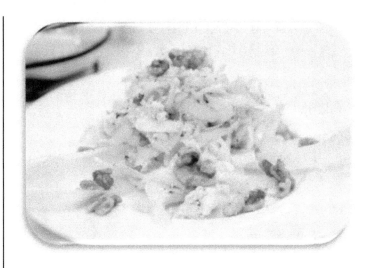

Ingredients:

- ½ cup walnut halves
- 1 Tbsp extra-virgin olive oil
- 1 tsp Dijon mustard
- 1 tsp red wine vinegar
- 4 heads Belgian endive (1 pound), cut lengthwise into long, thin strips
- ¼ tsp salt
- ⅛ tsp freshly ground black pepper

Instructions:

1. Heat the oven to 350°F. Spread walnuts on a baking sheet and toast for 10 minutes.
2. In a large bowl, whisk oil, mustard, and vinegar. Add the remaining ingredients to the bowl with dressing; toss to combine. Divide salad among 4 salad plates and serve.

Honeydew, Fresh Herb, and Ricotta Salata Salad (Phase II)

Prep time: 10 minutes

Cooking time: none

Servings: 4

Nutrients per serving:

Carbohydrates – 20 g

Fat – 8 g

Protein – 4 g

Calories – 160

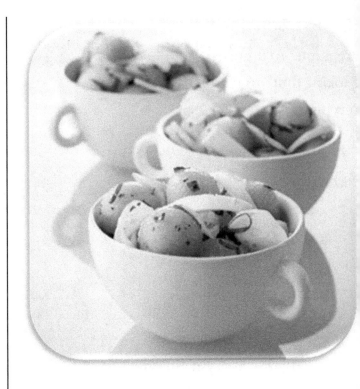

Ingredients:

- 1 (4- to 5-pound) honeydew melon, scooped into balls (4 cups)
- 1 cucumber, peeled, seeded and thinly sliced
- 1 Tbsp plus 1 tsp extra-virgin olive oil
- 1½ tsp red wine vinegar
- ¼ tsp salt
- ⅛ tsp freshly ground black pepper
- ¼ cup packed basil leaves, sliced
- 2 Tbsp chopped fresh parsley
- 2 ounces ricotta salata cheese

Instructions:

1. In a bowl, combine melon and cucumber. In another bowl, whisk together oil, vinegar, salt, and pepper; pour over melon and cucumber and toss to coat. Add basil and parsley and toss to combine. Divide salad among 4 bowls, cups, or plates, shave cheese over the top and serve.

Crisp Jícama Salad with Creamy Cilantro Dressing (Phase I)

Prep time: 15 minutes

Cooking time: none

Servings: 4

Nutrients per serving:

Carbohydrates – 13 g

Fat – 7 g

Protein – 4 g

Calories – 130

Ingredients:

- ½ cup low-fat plain yogurt
- ¼ cup finely chopped fresh cilantro
- 3 Tbsp fresh lime juice
- 2 Tbsp extra-virgin olive oil
- ¼ tsp salt
- ⅛ tsp freshly ground black pepper
- 1 (10-ounce) head red leaf lettuce, chopped (6 cups)
- 1 (1-pound) jícama, peeled and cut into matchsticks
- 1 medium cucumber, seeded and thinly sliced

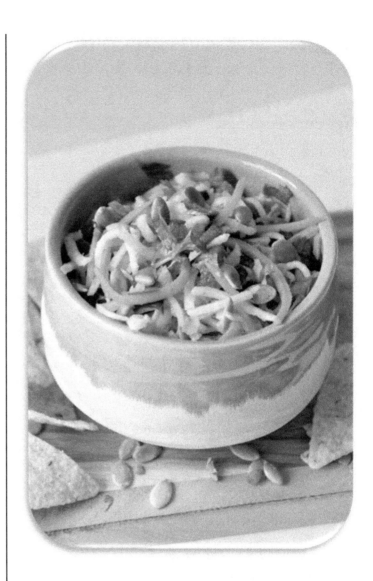

Instructions:

1. In a bowl, combine yogurt, cilantro, lime juice, oil, salt, and pepper. Place lettuce in a salad bowl and toss with ¼ cup of the dressing; divide among 4 salad plates. Add jícama and cucumber to the same salad bowl and toss with remaining dressing. Spoon jícama and cucumber mixture on top of lettuce and serve.

Romaine Hearts with Tuna, Edamame, and Green Goddess Dressing (Phase I)

Prep time: 10 minutes

Cooking time: none

Servings: 4

Nutrients per serving:

Carbohydrates – 9 g

Fat – 15 g

Protein – 27 g

Calories – 280

Ingredients:

- ½ medium avocado
- 3 Tbsp mayonnaise
- 3 Tbsp nonfat or low-fat plain yogurt
- 1 Tbsp water
- 2 scallions, chopped
- 1 small garlic clove
- 2 Tbsp chopped fresh basil
- 1 Tbsp chopped fresh parsley
- 1 Tbsp chopped fresh tarragon
- 2 tsp fresh lemon juice
- ¼ tsp salt
- ⅛ tsp freshly ground black pepper
- 3 romaine hearts, chopped (8 cups)
- 2 (6-ounce) cans water-packed chunk light tuna, drained and flaked
- 1 cup frozen shelled edamame, defrosted

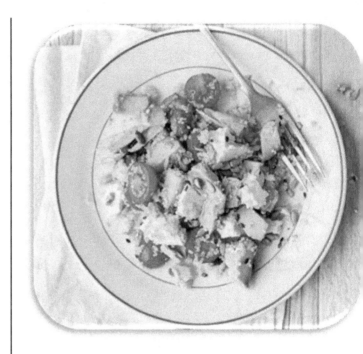

Instructions:

1. In a blender, combine avocado, mayonnaise, yogurt, water, scallions, and garlic; purée until smooth. Add basil, parsley, tarragon, lemon juice, salt, and pepper; blend just until combined.
2. In a large bowl, combine romaine, tuna, and edamame. Add dressing and toss. Serve at room temperature.

Baby Greens with Tiny Tomatoes, Fresh Herbs, and Toasted Pistachios (Phase I)

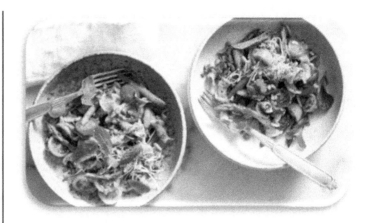

Prep time: 15 minutes

Cooking time: 8 minutes

Servings: 4

Nutrients per serving:

Carbohydrates – 13 g

Fat – 11 g

Protein – 6 g

Calories – 160

Ingredients:

- ½ cup unsalted shelled pistachios
- 6 ounces mixed baby greens (6 cups)
- 1½ cups cherry tomatoes, halved
- 1 medium cucumber, thinly sliced
- ¼ cup basil leaves, roughly chopped
- ¼ cup mint leaves, roughly chopped
- 1 Tbsp extra-virgin olive oil
- 2 tsp sherry vinegar
- ¼ tsp salt
- ⅛ tsp freshly ground black pepper

Instructions:

1. Heat the oven to 350°F. Toast pistachios for about 8 minutes on a baking sheet. Transfer to a cutting board and roughly chop.
2. In a bowl, combine all ingredients except pistachios; toss to coat. Divide salad among 4 plates, sprinkle with pistachios and serve.

Summertime Sweet Potato Salad (Phase II)

Prep time: 15 minutes

Cooking time: 20 minutes

Servings: 4

Nutrients per serving:

Carbohydrates – 27 g

Fat – 0 g

Protein – 4 g

Calories – 120

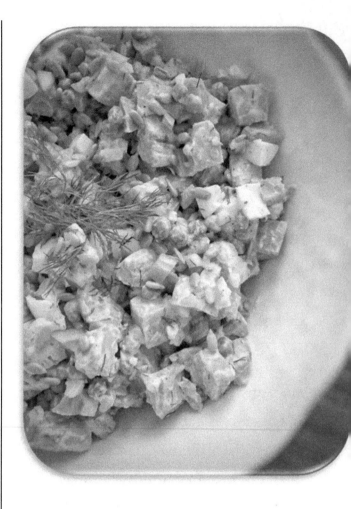

Ingredients:

- medium sweet potatoes (1 ½ pound), peeled, cut into 1-inch cubes
- ⅓ cup nonfat or low-fat plain yogurt
- 1 small red bell pepper, diced
- scallions, thinly sliced
- Tbsp chopped fresh basil
- 1 tsp red wine vinegar
- ¼ tsp salt
- ⅛ tsp freshly ground black pepper

Instructions:

1. In a medium saucepan, bring sweet potatoes to a boil and cook until tender, 8 to 10 minutes. Drain, run under cold water to cool.
2. In a large bowl, combine all ingredients. Serve at room temperature or chilled.

Savoy Slaw with Sesame Dressing (Phase I)

Prep time: 10 minutes

Cooking time: 5 minutes

Servings: 4

Nutrients per serving:

Carbohydrates – 7 g

Fat – 4.5 g

Protein – 2 g

Calories – 70

Ingredients:

- 1 Tbsp sesame seeds
- 1 (1½-pound) Savoy cabbage, shredded (4 cups)
- 1 red bell pepper, cut into thin strips
- 1 Tbsp toasted sesame oil
- 2 tsp red wine vinegar
- ¼ tsp salt
- ⅛ tsp freshly ground black pepper

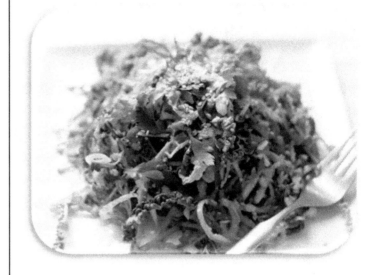

Instructions:

1. In a skillet, toast sesame seeds over medium-low heat, shaking the pan occasionally, until seeds are golden, about 5 minutes. Remove from the heat.
2. In a bowl, combine cabbage, bell pepper, sesame oil, vinegar, salt, and black pepper. Add sesame seeds and toss. Serve at room temperature.

Spanish Rice Salad with Pumpkin Seeds (Phase I)

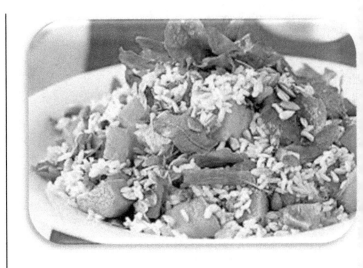

Prep time: 15 minutes

Cooking time: 15 minutes

Servings: 4

Nutrients per serving:

Carbohydrates – 25 g

Fat – 7 g

Protein – 4 g

Calories – 170

Ingredients:

- ½ cup quick-cooking whole-grain brown rice
- 2 medium tomatoes, chopped
- 1 small onion, chopped
- ½ cup pitted green olives, sliced lengthwise
- ¼ cup pumpkin seeds
- 1 Tbsp extra-virgin olive oil
- 1 tsp sherry vinegar
- 1 tsp dried oregano
- ¼ tsp salt
- ⅛ tsp freshly ground black pepper
- 2 Tbsp chopped fresh parsley

Instructions:

1. Cook rice according to package directions. Remove from the heat, spread on a plate, and refrigerate until cooled to room temperature, about 5 minutes.
2. In a bowl, combine rice, tomatoes, onion, olives, pumpkin seeds, oil, vinegar, oregano, salt, and pepper. Mix well and divide salad among 4 plates. Sprinkle with parsley just before serving.

DINNER

Garlicky Chicken Skewers (Phase I)

Prep time: 15 minutes

Cooking time: 10 minutes

Servings: 4

Nutrients per serving:

Carbohydrates – 11 g

Fat – 6 g

Protein – 42 g

Calories – 260

Ingredients:

- 1½ pounds chicken breasts, boneless, skinless, cut into 1-inch pieces
- 3 garlic cloves, finely minced
- 2 tsp dried rosemary
- 3 tsp extra-virgin olive oil
- Salt
- Freshly ground black pepper
- 1 small eggplant (1 pound), peeled and cut into ½-inch cubes
- 3 small zucchini, cut into ½-inch-thick rounds

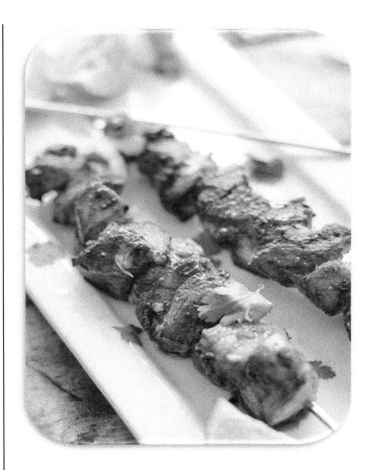

Instructions:

1. Coat a grill with cooking spray and heat to medium-high. In a medium bowl, combine chicken, garlic, rosemary, 2 tsp of the oil, ¼ tsp salt, and ⅛ tsp pepper; stir to coat well. Thread equal amounts of chicken onto 4 skewers.

2. In the same bowl, toss eggplant and zucchini pieces with remaining 1 tsp oil. Thread eggplant and zucchini pieces evenly onto 4 additional skewers. Lightly season with salt and pepper.

3. Grill chicken and vegetable skewers, turning every 2 minutes for about 8 minutes for chicken and 10 minutes for vegetables. Serve warm.

Turkey Cutlets with Vegetable Couscous (Phase II)

Prep time: 20 minutes

Cooking time: 15 minutes

Servings: 4

Nutrients per serving:

Carbohydrates – 16 g

Fat – 7 g

Protein – 45 g

Calories – 310

Ingredients:

- 1½ pounds turkey cutlets
- 3 garlic cloves, minced
- 3 Tbsp chopped fresh parsley
- 1 Tbsp plus 2 tsp extra-virgin olive oil
- 2 tsp finely grated lemon zest
- ⅛ tsp red pepper flakes
- 1 small yellow bell pepper, finely chopped
- 1 cup cherry tomatoes, halved
- 1 small cucumber, peeled and cut into ¼-inch cubes
- 1 Tbsp minced red onion
- 1 Tbsp red wine vinegar
- ¼ tsp salt
- ½ cup whole-wheat couscous

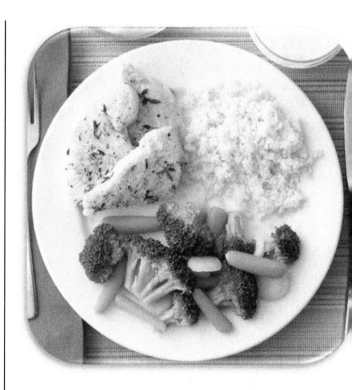

Instructions:

1. In a resealable plastic bag, combine turkey, garlic, parsley, 1 Tbsp of the oil, lemon zest, and pepper flakes; turn to coat well. Marinate for 15 minutes or refrigerate overnight.
2. While turkey is marinating, in a large bowl combine remaining 2 tsp oil, bell pepper, tomatoes, cucumber, onion, vinegar, and salt.
3. Prepare couscous according to package directions. Add hot couscous to vegetable mixture and stir well; keep warm.
4. Coat a nonstick skillet with cooking spray and heat. Add turkey and marinade to the skillet and cook on medium until cooked through, about 2 minutes per side. Serve warm with vegetable couscous.

Jerk Chicken with Cool Romaine Salad (Phase I)

Prep time: 20 minutes

Cooking time: 12 minutes

Servings: 4

Nutrients per serving:

Carbohydrates – 8 g

Fat – 3.5 g

Protein – 42 g

Calories – 230

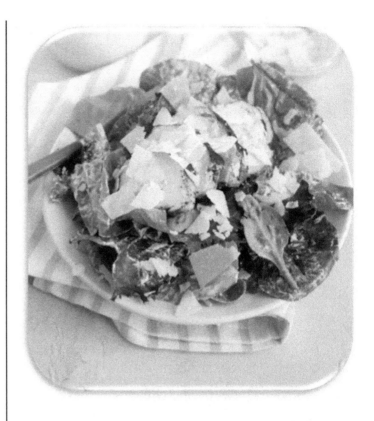

Ingredients:

- 1½ pounds boneless, skinless chicken breasts
- 1 Tbsp jerk seasoning
- 2 Tbsp reduced-fat sour cream
- 1 Tbsp fresh lime juice
- 1 (1-pound) head romaine lettuce, chopped (8 cups)
- 1 large cucumber, peeled and sliced
- 2 large plum tomatoes, chopped
- 2 scallions, chopped
- ¼ tsp salt

Instructions:

1. Pound chicken breasts to an even ½-inch thickness. Lightly rub jerk seasoning on both sides of chicken breasts. Refrigerate for at least 1 hour.
2. Coat a nonstick skillet with cooking spray. Add chicken and cook for about 5 minutes per side. Let rest for 5 minutes, then cut into ½-inch thick slices.
3. In a bowl, mix sour cream and lime juice. Add lettuce, cucumber, tomatoes, scallions, and salt; toss well. Place salad equally on 4 plates, top with chicken slices, and serve warm.

Grilled Pork Tenderloin with Peach-Lime Salsa (Phase II)

Prep time: 15 minutes

Cooking time: 30 minutes

Servings: 4

Nutrients per serving:

Carbohydrates – 12 g

Fat – 8 g

Protein – 37 g

Calories – 270

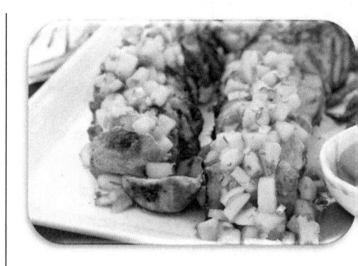

Ingredients:

- 2 garlic cloves, minced
- 2 tsp extra-virgin olive oil
- ¼ tsp freshly ground black pepper
- 1½ pounds pork tenderloin
- 2 peaches, peeled and cut into ½-inch pieces
- 1 small red onion, minced
- ¼ cup finely chopped fresh mint
- 3 Tbsp fresh lime juice
- ¼ tsp salt

Instructions:

1. In a bowl, combine garlic, oil, and pepper to form a rough paste. Place pork in a 9-by-13-inch glass baking dish and coat with garlic paste; let stand at room temperature for 10 minutes.
2. In another small bowl combine the rest of ingredients.
3. Coat a grill with cooking spray and heat to medium-high. Grill pork 12 to 14 minutes per side, or until a thermometer inserted into the thickest part reads 150°F to 155°F. Let rest for 5 to 10 minutes.
4. Slice pork into 1 /2-inch-thick slices and serve warm with peach-lime salsa.

Carne Asada (Phase I)

Prep time: 15 minutes

Cooking time: 25 minutes

Servings: 4

Nutrients per serving:

Carbohydrates – 13 g

Fat – 17 g

Protein – 38 g

Calories – 360

Ingredients:

- ¼ cup fresh lime juice
- 2 garlic cloves, minced
- ½ tsp freshly ground black pepper
- ⅛ tsp salt
- 1 (1½-pound) flank steak, about 1 inch thick
- 1 large red onion, sliced into ¼-inch-thick rounds
- ½ tsp extra-virgin olive oil
- 1 small avocado, sliced into ¼-inch-thick pieces
- 1 cup fresh tomato salsa

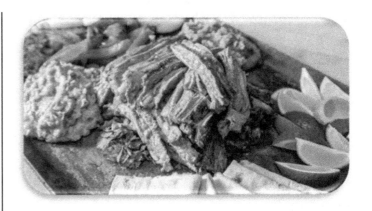

Instructions:

1. In a 9- by 13-inch glass baking dish, combine lime juice, garlic, pepper, and salt. Add steak and turn to coat. Marinate steak for 20 minutes.
2. Coat a grill with cooking spray. Grill steak on medium, basting with any remaining marinade, 5 to 7 minutes per side for medium-rare. Let rest for 5 to 10 minutes.
3. In a bowl toss onion with oil. Grill the onion, turning occasionally, until golden, 4 to 5 minutes. Slice steak and divide among 4 plates. Serve with onion, avocado, and salsa.

Kofta Skewers with Peppers (Phase I)

Prep time: 20 minutes

Cooking time: 17 minutes

Servings: 4

Nutrients per serving:

Carbohydrates – 8 g

Fat – 21 g

Protein – 35 g

Calories – 360

Ingredients:

- 1 pound extra-lean ground beef
- ½ pound lean ground lamb
- 1 small onion, grated
- ¼ cup chopped fresh parsley
- 2 Tbsp tomato paste
- 2 garlic cloves, minced
- 1 Tbsp ground cumin
- 1 tsp red pepper flakes
- ¼ tsp salt
- 2 medium bell peppers, cut into ½-inch-wide strips
- 1 tsp extra-virgin olive oil

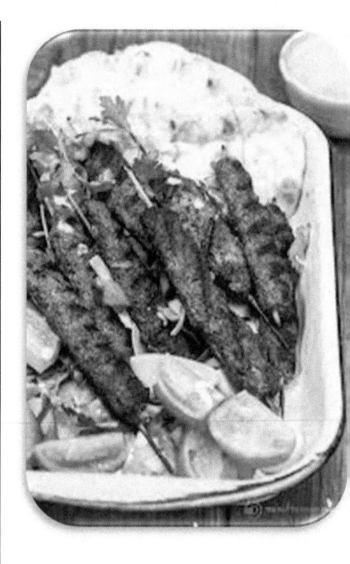

Instructions:

1. In a large bowl, combine first nine ingredients. Divide meat mixture into 8 equal portions. Form each portion into a 6-inch sausage shape around a skewer.
2. In a medium bowl, toss peppers with oil.
3. Coat a grill with cooking spray. Grill meat for about 15 minutes. Halfway through cooking, place peppers on the grill and cook for 8 to 10 minutes. Serve kofta hot with peppers.

Spice-Rubbed Grilled Pork Chops (Phase II)

Prep time: 10 minutes

Cooking time: 2 minutes

Servings: 4

Nutrients per serving:

Carbohydrates – 0 g

Fat – 14 g

Protein – 32 g

Calories – 265

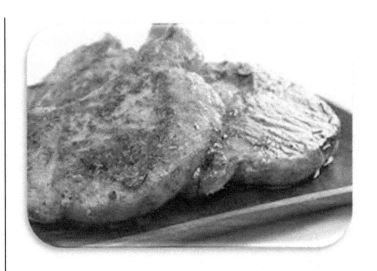

Ingredients:

- 1 tsp ground coriander
- ½ tsp ground cumin
- ½ tsp garam masala
- ½ tsp smoked paprika
- ¼ tsp dried oregano, crumbled
- ¼ tsp salt
- ¼ tsp freshly ground black pepper
- ⅛ tsp garlic powder
- 8 boneless pork loin chops (3 ounces each)
- 1 Tbsp extra-virgin olive oil

Instructions:

1. In a small bowl, stir together the coriander, cumin, garam masala, paprika, oregano, salt, pepper, and garlic powder.
2. Coat a grill or grill pan with cooking spray and heat over medium heat.
3. Sprinkle each side of each pork chop with a little more than ¼ teaspoon of the rub. Rub with oil. Grill the pork for 1 to 1½ minutes per side.

Chicken with Lemon-Scallion Sauce (Phase II)

Prep time: 15 minutes

Cooking time: 10 minutes

Servings: 4

Nutrients per serving:

Carbohydrates – 5 g

Fat – 9.5 g

Protein – 38 g

Calories – 263

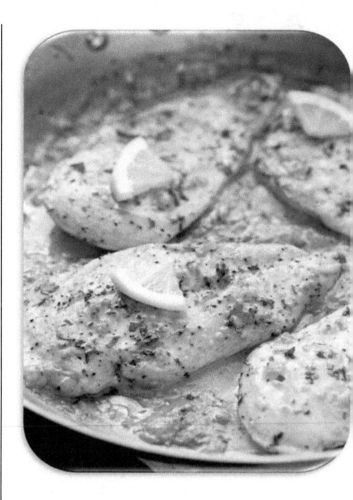

Ingredients:

- 1¼ cups reduced-sodium gluten-free chicken broth
- 3 Tbsp chickpea flour
- 2 tsp grated lemon zest
- ¼ cup fresh lemon juice
- ¼ tsp garlic powder
- ¼ tsp salt
- ¼ tsp freshly ground black pepper
- 4 tsp extra-virgin olive oil
- 1½ pounds boneless, skinless chicken breasts
- 6 scallions, chopped
- 2 Tbsp minced fresh cilantro or parsley

Instructions:

1. In a small bowl, stir ½ cup of the chicken broth into the chickpea flour to make a smooth paste. Then stir in the remaining ¾ cup chicken broth, the lemon zest, lemon juice, garlic powder, salt, and pepper. Stir well to blend. Set aside.

2. In a large nonstick skillet, heat 2 tsp of the oil over medium-high heat. Add the chicken and cook about 5 minutes.

3. Transfer the chicken to a plate.

4. Add 2 tsp oil and the scallions to the skillet and stir until beginning to soften about 1 minute. Stir the chicken broth mixture to recombine and pour the mixture into the skillet. Bring to a boil, stirring, then stir the cilantro or parsley into the sauce.

5. Return the chicken (and the collected juices on the plate) to the skillet, toss to coat with the sauce, and cook to heat through about 45 seconds.

Sliced Beef with Bell Pepper, Onion, and Snow Peas (Phase II)

Prep time: 20 minutes

Cooking time: 20 minutes

Servings: 4

Nutrients per serving:

Carbohydrates – 8 g

Fat – 15 g

Protein – 40 g

Calories – 333

Ingredients:

- 1½ pounds top round steak (about ¾ inch thick), well trimmed
- Salt
- Freshly ground black pepper
- 1 tsp extra-virgin olive oil
- 1 large green bell pepper, thinly sliced
- 1 medium onion, thinly sliced
- 1 garlic clove, minced
- 6 ounces snow peas, strings removed, thinly sliced
- 2 Tbsp water
- 1 Tbsp low-sodium soy sauce

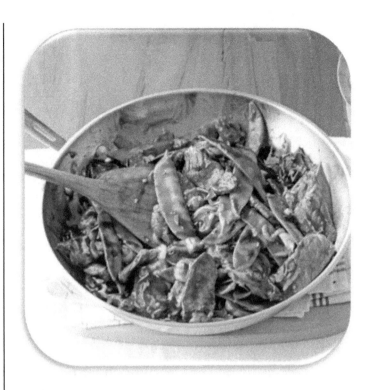

Instructions:

1. Season steak with salt and black pepper. Coat a large nonstick skillet with cooking spray. Add steak and cook on medium for 4 minutes per side for medium-rare; remove from heat. Let sit for 5 minutes before slicing.

2. Meanwhile, in the same skillet, heat oil. Add bell pepper, onion, and garlic; cook, stirring constantly, 5 minutes. Add peas and water. Cook covered for 5 minutes. Add soy sauce, and cook 30 seconds longer. Add sliced steak to skillet and toss briefly, just to heat through. Serve warm.

Tomato-Saffron Stewed Chicken (Phase II)

Prep time: 10 minutes

Cooking time: 30 minutes

Servings: 4

Nutrients per serving:

Carbohydrates – 13 g

Fat – 9 g

Protein – 41 g

Calories – 300

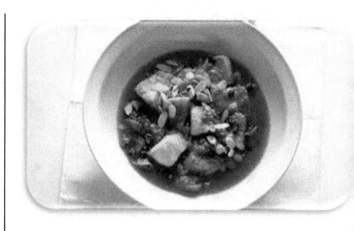

Ingredients:

- (6-ounce) boneless, skinless chicken breasts, cut in half crosswise on the diagonal
- 2 Tbsp extra-virgin olive oil
- 1 medium onion, thinly sliced
- 2 garlic cloves, minced
- 1 (28-ounce) can unsalted diced tomatoes
- ¼ tsp powdered saffron
- ¼ cup fresh parsley leaves, roughly chopped
- Salt and freshly ground black pepper

Instructions:

1. Season chicken with salt and pepper. Heat oil in a large saucepan. Add chicken and cook for about 3 minutes per side. Remove chicken from pan.
2. Add onion and garlic to the same saucepan and cook over medium-high heat for 2 minutes. Return chicken to the pan, add tomatoes with juice and saffron, bring to a low boil, reduce to a simmer, and cook for 15 minutes. Stir in parsley, season with salt and pepper, and serve.

Chicken Piri-Piri (Phase I)

Prep time: 20 minutes

Cooking time: 10 minutes

Servings: 4

Nutrients per serving:

Carbohydrates – 1 g

Fat – 16 g

Protein – 39 g

Calories – 310

Ingredients:

- ¼ cup extra-virgin olive oil
- 2 Tbsp cider vinegar
- 1 jalapeño pepper, seeded and minced
- 1 garlic clove, minced
- ¼ tsp red pepper flakes
- ¼ tsp salt
- 4 (6-ounce) boneless, skinless chicken breasts

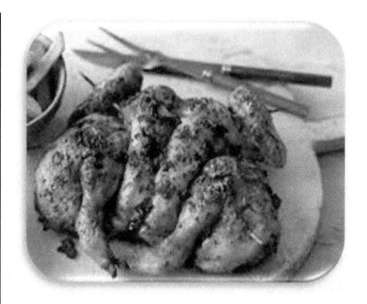

Instructions:

1. Heat a grill or grill pan to high.
2. Whisk together oil, vinegar, jalapeño, garlic, red pepper flakes, and salt in a small bowl. Place chicken in a shallow dish. Add 3 Tbsp of the marinade and turn to coat. Let stand at room temperature 10 minutes.
3. Grill chicken, turning often, until juices run clear, about 10 minutes. Drizzle with remaining sauce (do not use the leftover marinade that the chicken was in) and serve.

Peanut Chicken with Noodles (Phase II)

Prep time: 15 minutes

Cooking time: 20 minutes

Servings: 4

Nutrients per serving:

Carbohydrates – 19 g

Fat – 13 g

Protein – 42 g

Calories – 370

Ingredients:

- 4 ounces soba noodles
- 1½ pounds boneless, skinless chicken breasts
- 3 tsp dark sesame oil, divided
- ⅓ cup creamy trans-fat-free peanut butter
- 2 Tbsp low-sodium soy sauce
- 2 Tbsp rice vinegar
- 2 Tbsp water
- 1 (¾-pound) head napa cabbage, shredded (4 cups)
- 2 scallions, thinly sliced
- Salt and freshly ground black pepper

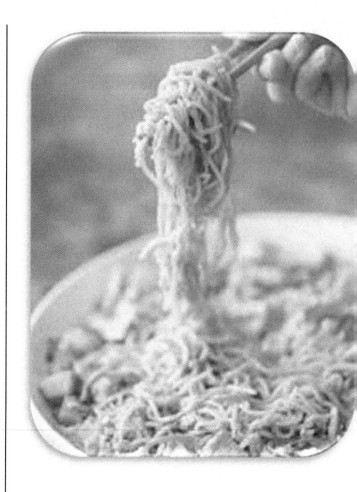

Instructions:

1. Cook noodles according to package directions.
2. Season chicken with salt and pepper and toss with 1 tsp of the oil. Heat a grill pan or a skillet over medium-high heat; cook chicken until browned and cooked through, about 4 minutes per side. Transfer to a cutting board.
3. In a mixing bowl, whisk together peanut butter, soy sauce, vinegar, water, and remaining oil. Slice chicken and add to peanut butter mixture. Add the noodles, raw cabbage, and scallions; toss to combine and serve.

Chicken Couscous (Phase II)

Prep time: 15 minutes

Cooking time: 15 minutes

Servings: 4

Nutrients per serving:

Carbohydrates – 32 g

Fat – 6 g

Protein – 33 g

Calories – 320

Ingredients:

- 1 pound boneless, skinless chicken breasts, cut into ¾-inch cubes
- 1 Tbsp extra-virgin olive oil
- 1 small onion, diced
- ½ tsp ground cumin
- ¼ tsp ground cinnamon
- 1 cup low-sodium chicken broth
- ½ cup whole-wheat couscous
- 1 (15-ounce) can chickpeas, rinsed and drained
- Salt and freshly ground black pepper

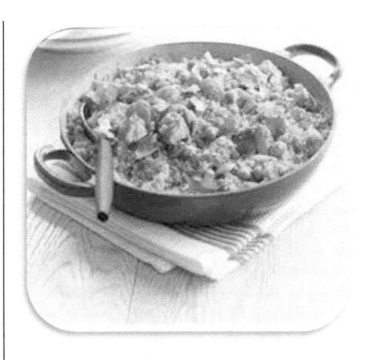

Instructions:

1. Season chicken with salt and pepper. Heat oil in a saucepan. Cook chicken for about 6 minutes. Remove chicken from pan with and drain on paper towels.

2. Reduce heat to medium and add onion, cumin, and cinnamon to the same pan; cook until onions are softened and lightly browned, about 3 minutes. Add broth and bring to a simmer. Stir in couscous, chickpeas, and a good pinch of salt and pepper. Cook covered on low for 3 minutes. Return chicken to saucepan, mix with the couscous, season to taste with salt and pepper, and serve.

Rosemary Pork Medallions with Chunky Applesauce (Phase II)

Prep time: 5 minutes

Cooking time: 25 minutes

Servings: 4

Nutrients per serving:

Carbohydrates – 24 g

Fat – 13 g

Protein – 3 g

Calories – 360

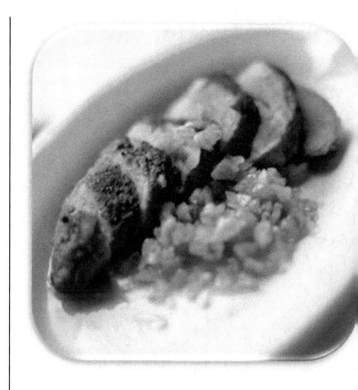

Ingredients:

- 3 tsp extra-virgin olive oil, divided
- 1 small onion, diced
- 3 McIntosh apples (or other sweet variety), peeled, cored, and diced
- 1 Tbsp balsamic vinegar
- 3 Tbsp water
- 1½ pounds pork tenderloin, cut into medallions, about ¾ inch thick
- 2 tsp dried rosemary
- Salt and freshly ground black pepper

Instructions:

1. Heat 2 tsp of the oil in a skillet over medium heat. Add onion and cook for about 3 minutes. Add apples, vinegar, and water; reduce heat to low and cook until tender, about 10 minutes. Remove from heat.
2. Season pork with rosemary, salt, and pepper. Heat remaining oil in a nonstick skillet. Add pork and cook for about 4 minutes per side; remove from pan and serve with applesauce.

DESSERTS

Lemon Polenta Cake
(Phase II)

Prep time: 15 minutes

Cooking time: 30 minutes

Servings: 10

Nutrients per serving:

Carbohydrates – 15 g

Fat – 12 g

Protein – 4 g

Calories – 175

Ingredients:

- Olive oil cooking spray
- ½ cup regular cornmeal (not stone-ground), plus more for dusting
- ¾ cup almond flour
- 1 tsp gluten-free baking powder
- ¼ tsp baking soda
- ¼ tsp salt
- 1 tsp grated lemon zest
- 1 large egg
- ⅓ cup liquid egg whites (or the whites of 2 large eggs)
- ⅓ cup light (1.5%) buttermilk
- ⅓ cup extra-virgin olive oil
- 3 Tbsp agave nectar
- ½ cup granulated stevia (baking formula)
- ½ tsp dried crumbled rosemary

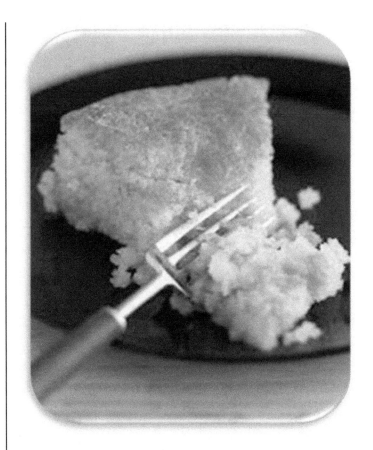

Instructions:

1. Preheat the oven to 375°F. Coat an 8-inch round cake pan with olive oil cooking spray and dust it with cornmeal. In a bowl, whisk together the cornmeal, almond flour, baking powder, baking soda, salt, and lemon zest.

2. In another large bowl, whisk together the whole egg, egg whites, buttermilk, oil, agave nectar, stevia, and rosemary. Combine dry and egg mixtures. Pour into the cake pan and bake for 25 to 30 minutes.

3. Let cool for 15 minutes in the pan, then run a spatula around the edges of the pan and invert the cake onto a rack. Cut into 10 wedges. Serve warm or at room temperature.

Pistachio Biscotti (Phase II)

Prep time: 20 minutes

Cooking time: 30 minutes

Servings: 10

Nutrients per serving:

Carbohydrates – 3 g

Fat – 4.5 g

Protein – 2 g

Calories – 54

Ingredients:

- ⅓ cups almond flour
- ¼ cup granulated stevia (baking formula)
- ½ tsp xanthan gum
- ¼ tsp baking soda
- ¼ tsp salt
- 1 tsp grated lime zest
- ¾ tsp ground cinnamon
- 1 Tbsp plus 1 tsp fresh lime juice
- ⅓ cup liquid egg whites (or the whites of 2 large eggs)
- ¼ cup pistachios, chopped

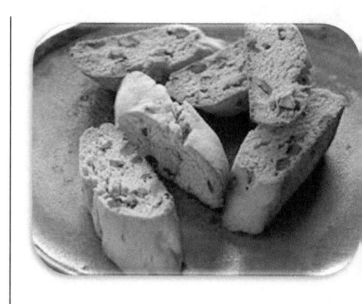

Instructions:

1. Preheat the oven to 350°F. Line a baking sheet with parchment paper.
2. In a food processor, pulse the almond flour, stevia, xanthan gum, baking soda, salt, lime zest, and cinnamon. Add the lime juice and egg whites and pulse until the dough forms a ball. Transfer to a bowl and knead in the pistachios.
3. Divide the dough in and shape each part into a log 6½ inches long, 2½ inches wide, and ½ inch thick. Place the two logs on the baking sheet, spacing them 2 inches apart. Bake until firmed and set about 20 minutes. Remove from the oven reduce the oven temperature to 300°F.
4. Let the logs cool slightly on a rack. Then slice each log crosswise into 10 biscotti. Return the cookies to the baking sheet, laying them flat, and bake until crisp, about 10 minutes. Transfer to a rack to cool.

Banana-Nut Snack Bars
(Phase II)

Prep time: 20 minutes

Cooking time: 30 minutes

Servings: 10

Nutrients per serving:

Carbohydrates – 23 g

Fat – 6 g

Protein – 3 g

Calories – 150

Ingredients:

- 1 cup gluten-free rolled oats
- ½ cup pecans
- ⅓ cup (½ ounce) unsweetened, gluten-free dried apple slices, broken into
- small bits
- 3 Tbsp gluten-free dried currants
- 3 Tbsp ground flaxmeal
- ¼ tsp salt
- ¾ cup mashed banana (from 2 medium bananas)
- 3 Tbsp agave nectar
- 3 Tbsp liquid egg whites (or the white of 1 large egg)
- 1 tsp pure vanilla extract

Instructions:

1. Preheat the oven to 350°F. Place the oats in a baking pan and bake until fragrant and lightly browned, about 10 minutes. Leave the oven on.

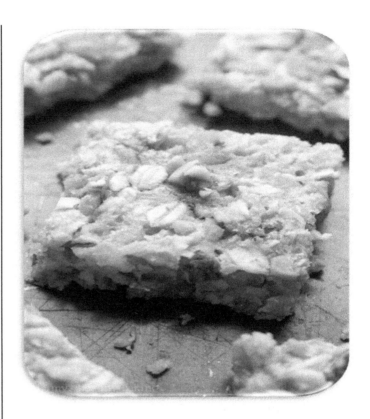

2. Meanwhile, coat an 8 × 8-inch baking pan with cooking spray. Line the pan with parchment, coat the parchment with cooking spray.

3. Transfer ½ cup of the toasted oats to a large bowl. Coarsely chop ¼ cup of the pecans and add them to the bowl along with the dried apple, currants, flaxmeal, and salt. In a food processor, grind ½ cup toasted oats and the remaining ¼ cup pecans. Add them to the bowl along with the mashed banana, agave nectar, egg whites, and vanilla. Stir to combine.

4. Spoon the mixture into the baking pan and pat to an even layer. Bake until set, about 20 minutes. Let cool in the pan. Lift the baked snack from the pan using the parchment ends and cut into 10 bars.

Mango Lassi (Phase II)

Prep time: 10 minutes

Cooking time: none

Servings: 4

Nutrients per serving:

Carbohydrates – 15 g

Fat – 0.5 g

Protein – 4 g

Calories – 80

Ingredients:

- 1 mango, peeled and roughly chopped
- 1½ cups low-fat plain yogurt
- ½ cup chilled water
- 1 Tbsp granular sugar substitute
- Pinch ground cardamom (optional)
- Ice cubes

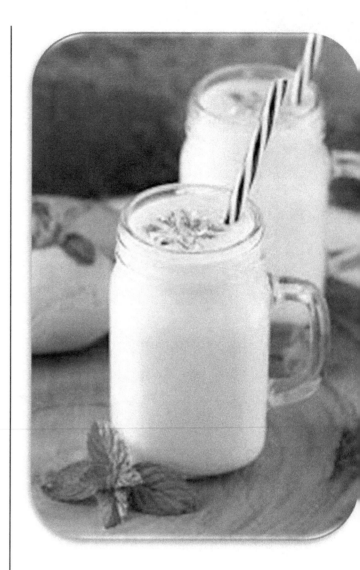

Instructions:

1. In a blender, combine mango, yogurt, water, sugar substitute, and cardamom, if using; purée until smooth. Fill 4 (8-ounce) glasses with ice cubes. Pour Mango Lassi over ice and serve.

Orange Gingerade (Phase II)

Prep time: 15 minutes

Cooking time: none

Servings: 4

Nutrients per serving:

Carbohydrates – 10 g

Fat – 0 g

Protein – 1 g

Calories – 40

Ingredients:

- 1½ cups water
- 4 ounces fresh ginger, peeled, chopped 2 seedless oranges, peeled and chopped
- Ice cubes
- 3 Tbsp granular sugar substitute

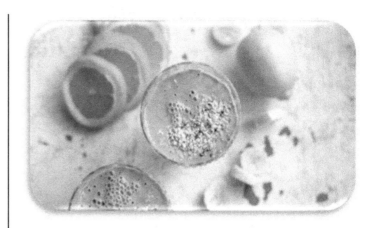

Instructions:

1. In a saucepan, bring water to a boil and remove from the heat. Add ginger and steep for 10 minutes. While ginger is steeping, purée oranges in a blender until smooth.

2. Strain steeped ginger water into a pitcher; discard ginger. Add 1 cup ice cubes and sugar substitute to ginger water and stir for about 3 minutes. Add puréed oranges and stir to combine.

3. Fill 4 glasses with ice cubes; pour Orange Gingerade over ice and serve.

Plum Rice Pudding (Phase II)

Prep time: 5 minutes

Cooking time: 10 minutes

Servings: 4

Nutrients per serving:

Carbohydrates – 39 g

Fat – 0.5 g

Protein – 6 g

Calories – 210

Ingredients:

- 1 Tbsp slivered almonds
- 2 cups cooked whole-grain brown rice
- 1¼ cups fat-free half-and-half plus 1 Tbsp
- 1 tsp granular sugar substitute
- 1 tsp vanilla extract
- 3 small plums, thinly sliced
- 1 tsp ground cinnamon

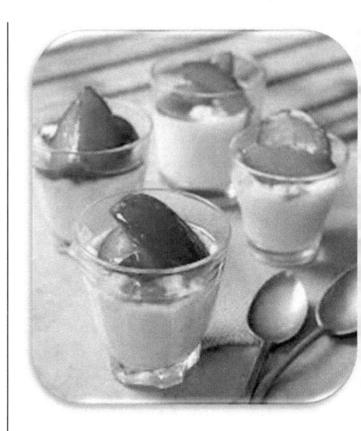

Instructions:

1. Heat the oven to 275°F. Toast almonds on a baking sheet, stirring once, for about 7 minutes. Transfer to a plate to cool.

2. While almonds are toasting, in a medium saucepan bring rice, half-and-half, sugar substitute, and vanilla to a simmer over medium heat, stirring occasionally. Add 2 plums and cinnamon; cook until liquid is absorbed and plums are softened about 8 minutes. Transfer pudding to 4 dessert bowls, top with remaining plum and serve hot.

Summer Fruit Cocktail (Phase II)

Prep time: 15 minutes

Cooking time: none

Servings: 4

Nutrients per serving:

Carbohydrates – 11 g

Fat – 0 g

Protein – 1 g

Calories – 45

Ingredients:

- 2 medium peaches, cubed
- ⅔ cup blueberries
- 5 medium strawberries, sliced
- 2 tsp fresh lemon juice
- 1 tsp granular sugar substitute
- 1 Tbsp sliced fresh mint

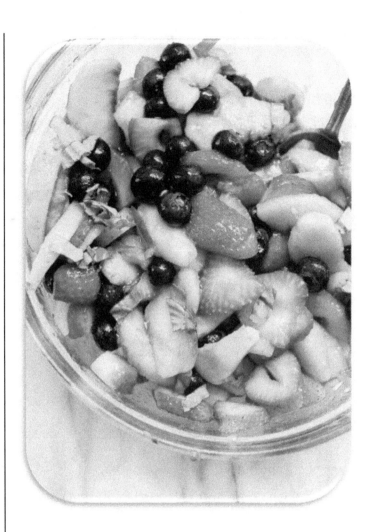

Instructions:

1. In a large bowl, gently combine peaches, blueberries, and strawberries. Add lemon juice and sugar substitute; toss gently. Divide fruit among 4 bowls, sprinkle with mint and serve.

Cool-Down-Quick Peach Pops (Phase II)

Prep time: 10 minutes

Cooking time: none

Servings: 4

Nutrients per serving:

Carbohydrates – 5 g

Fat – 0 g

Protein – 1 g

Calories – 20

Ingredients:

- medium peaches, peeled and cubed
- ½ cup water
- 2 Tbsp granular sugar substitute
- 1 cup nonfat or low-fat plain yogurt
- 2 Tbsp chopped fresh basil (optional)

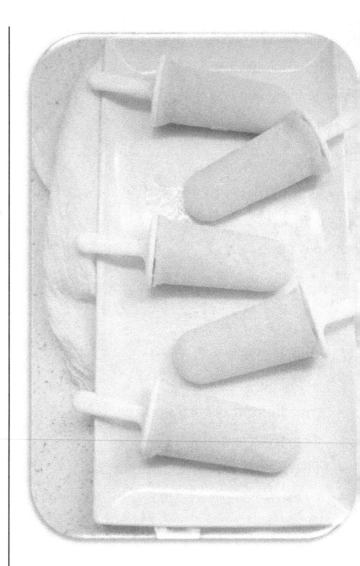

Instructions:

1. In a blender, purée peaches with water until smooth. Add sugar substitute, yogurt, and basil, if using, and blend until combined. Divide mixture evenly among paper cups or pop molds and insert a wooden stick into the center of each. Place pops in the freezer for 4 hours. Peel off paper cups, if using, serve.

Fresh Blackberry Tartlets (Phase II)

Prep time: 10 minutes

Cooking time: 5 minutes

Servings: 4

Nutrients per serving:

Carbohydrates – 13 g

Fat – 3 g

Protein – 2 g

Calories – 100

Ingredients:

- 12 frozen mini phyllo tart shells, thawed
- 15 blackberries
- ¾ cup fat-free or light whipped topping
- 1 tsp fresh lemon juice
- ¼ tsp vanilla extract

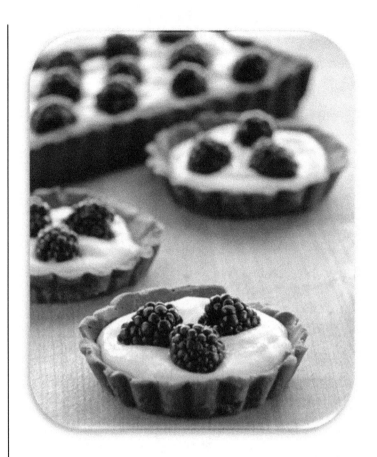

Instructions:

1. Heat the oven to 350°F. Bake tart shells on a baking sheet until crisp, 3 to 5 minutes. Allow cooling before filling, about 5 minutes.

2. Set aside 12 blackberries for topping the tarts. Place remaining blackberries in a small bowl and mash with a fork. Add whipped topping and stir to combine. Stir in lemon juice and vanilla.

3. Spoon 1 Tbsp of the whipped topping mixture into each tart shell. Top each tart with 3 blackberries and serve.

Baked Sweet Potato Chips (Phase II)

Prep time: 15 minutes

Cooking time: 17 minutes

Servings: 4

Nutrients per serving:

Carbohydrates – 46 g

Fat – 2 g

Protein – 4 g

Calories – 216

Ingredients:

- 2 large sweet potatoes (2 pounds), sliced into ¼-inch-thick round slices
- 2 tsp extra-virgin olive oil
- 1 Tbsp Italian seasoning
- Salt
- Freshly ground black pepper

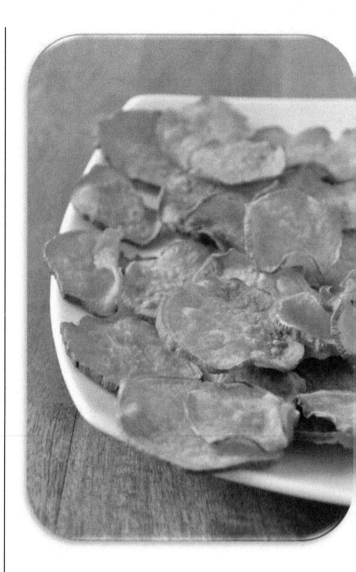

Instructions:

1. Heat the oven to 400°F.
2. In a bowl, toss potatoes with oil, Italian seasoning, and a pinch of salt and pepper. Spread on two baking sheets and bake for 10 minutes. Turn slices over and continue baking for about 7 minutes longer.
3. Serve warm.

Coconut Wafers (Phase II)

Prep time: 10 minutes

Cooking time: 24 minutes

Servings: 6

Nutrients per serving:

Carbohydrates – 12 g

Fat – 11 g

Protein – 2 g

Calories – 150

Ingredients:

- 2 large egg whites
- ⅛ tsp salt
- 2 Tbsp granular sugar substitute
- 2 Tbsp sugar
- ½ tsp vanilla extract
- 2 Tbsp whole-wheat flour
- ¾ cup unsweetened shredded coconut
- 2 Tbsp trans-fat-free margarine, melted

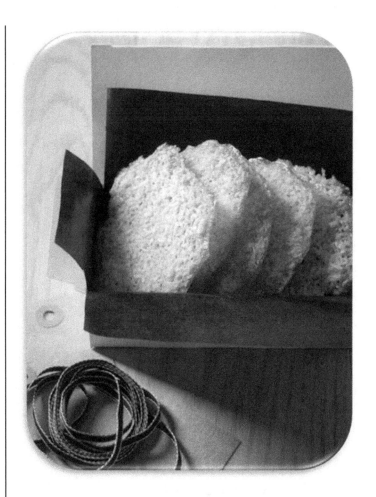

Instructions:

1. Heat oven to 350°F. Line a baking pan with foil and coat with cooking spray.
2. Whisk egg whites, salt, sugar substitute, sugar, and vanilla in a medium bowl until light and foamy, about 2 minutes. Sift in flour and stir to combine. Stir in coconut. Slowly whisk in margarine until incorporated.
3. Drop 6 (2-tsp) balls of batter onto the pan. Using a butter knife, spread each ball into a 3-inch disk. Bake until the edges are golden, about 12 minutes. Let cool completely. Repeat with the remaining batter. Serve.

Fruit Salad with Lime and Mint (Phase II)

Prep time: 10 minutes

Cooking time: none

Servings: 4

Nutrients per serving:

Carbohydrates – 23 g

Fat – 0 g

Protein – 1 g

Calories – 90

Ingredients:

- 3 cups honeydew melon balls
- 2 cups blueberries or blackberries, or a mix
- 1 heaping Tbsp chopped fresh mint
- 1 Tbsp fresh lime juice

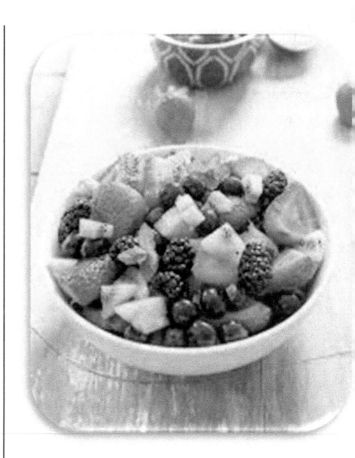

Instructions:

1. Place melon balls, berries, mint, and lime juice in a mixing bowl and toss to combine. Serve cold in bowls or martini glasses.

Sweet Cherries with Yogurt (Phase II)

Prep time: 5 minutes

Cooking time: none

Servings: 4

Nutrients per serving:

Carbohydrates – 34 g

Fat – 4 g

Protein – 10 g

Calories – 200

Ingredients:

- 1 (16-ounce) package fresh unsweetened Bing cherries
- 1 tsp grated lemon zest
- 2 Tbsp granular sugar substitute
- 24 ounces plain fat-free or low-fat yogurt

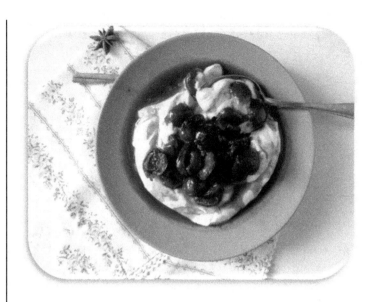

Instructions:

1. Bring cherries, lemon zest, and sugar substitute to a simmer in a small saucepan filled with water over medium-low heat. Cook, stirring occasionally until cherries have softened, about 5 minutes. Remove from heat and cool slightly.
2. Divide yogurt among 4 serving dishes. Top each serving with a ¼ cup of the cherries and serve.

Five Ingredients or Less

Melon Slush (Phase II)

Prep time: 5 minutes

Cooking time: none

Servings: 4

Nutrients per serving:

Carbohydrates – 17 g

Fat – 10 g

Protein – 5 g

Calories – 60

Ingredients:

- 12 ice cubes
- 4 cups cubed cantaloupe
- 1½ tsp fresh lemon juice
- 1½ tsp granular sugar substitute

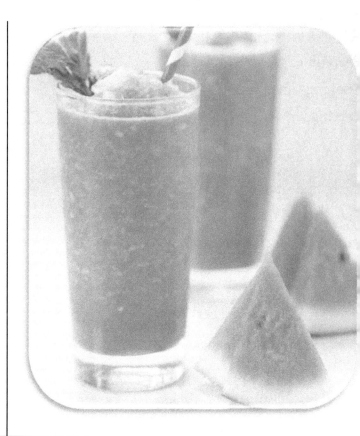

Instructions:

1. Place ice cubes in a blender and blend until crushed. Add remaining ingredients. Blend until combined, about 10 seconds. Serve immediately.

Mango Smoothie (Phase II)

Prep time: 10 minutes

Cooking time: none

Servings: 4

Nutrients per serving:

Carbohydrates – 30 g

Fat – 0 g

Protein – 4 g

Calories – 140

Ingredients:

- 2 mangoes, peeled, pitted, and diced
- 1½ cups sugar-free vanilla fat-free or low-fat yogurt
- Ice cubes

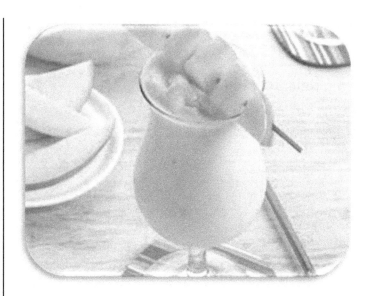

Instructions:

1. Purée mangoes in a blender. Add yogurt and 4 or 5 ice cubes; blend for about 30 seconds. Pour into glasses and serve.

Chipotle Chiles with Grilled Onions (Phase I)

Prep time: 10 minutes

Cooking time: 12 minutes

Servings: 4

Nutrients per serving:

Carbohydrates – 7 g

Fat – 0 g

Protein – 1 g

Calories – 30

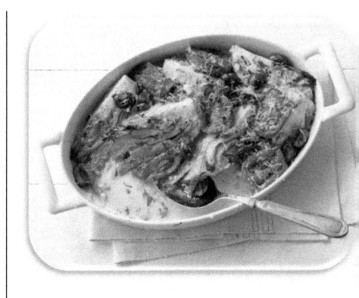

Ingredients:

- 2 onions, cut into ½-inch-thick rounds
- ¼ tsp salt
- ⅛ tsp freshly ground black pepper
- 2 canned chipotle chiles in adobo, rinsed, seeded, and minced
- 4 plum tomatoes, sliced
- 2 tsp fresh lime juice

Instructions:

1. Coat a grill with cooking spray and heat to medium-high.
2. In a medium bowl, toss onions (rings can be separate) and tomatoes with salt and pepper. Grill onions and tomatoes, turning occasionally until lightly browned 10 to 12 minutes. Return onions and tomatoes to the bowl, add chiles and lime juice and toss until the onions are well coated. Serve warm.

Stuffed Pork Burger (Phase I)

Prep time: 10 minutes

Cooking time: 10 minutes

Servings: 4

Nutrients per serving:

Carbohydrates – 1 g

Fat – 22 g

Protein – 42 g

Calories – 380

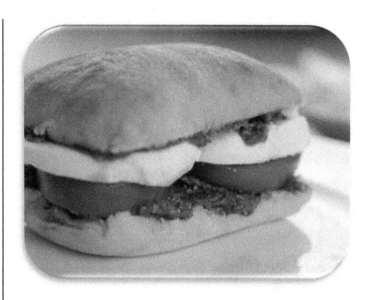

Ingredients:

- 5 Tbsp commercially prepared pesto
- Pepper, salt to taste
- 1½ pounds lean ground pork
- 1 large tomato, thickly sliced (4 slices)
- 2 ounces low-fat mozzarella, cut into 4 cubes

Instructions:

1. Mix the first three ingredients together in a mixing bowl. Add pork and, gently yet thoroughly, combine; do not overmix.

2. Shape pork mixture into 4 equal-sized balls. Press 1 mozzarella cube into the center of each ball; form a ¾-inch-thick patty, enclosing the cheese.

3. Coat a nonstick skillet with cooking spray. Add burgers, and brown quickly on each side. Reduce heat to medium, and cook 5 minutes per side. Serve hot on buns.

Peppery Steak with Horseradish Cream (Phase I)

Prep time: 5 minutes

Cooking time: 20 minutes

Servings: 4

Nutrients per serving:

Carbohydrates – 4 g

Fat – 18 g

Protein – 39 g

Calories – 360

Ingredients:

- 1½ pounds London broil or another sirloin steak (about 1 inch thick)
- 1 tsp extra-virgin olive oil
- 2 Tbsp cracked black pepper
- ½ cup reduced-fat sour cream
- 2 tsp prepared horseradish
- Salt

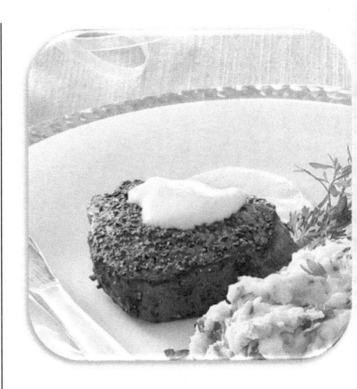

Instructions:

1. Rub steak with oil and pepper, pressing pepper into steak; season well with salt.
2. Heat a grill pan over medium-high heat or heat an oven on broil. Grill or broil steak 5 to 6 minutes per side for medium-rare. Let rest for 5 minutes. Slice thinly.
3. While steak is resting, mix together sour cream and horseradish; season to taste with salt. Serve horseradish cream with steak slices.

Baked Pesto Chicken (Phase I)

Prep time: 5 minutes

Cooking time: 30 minutes

Servings: 4

Nutrients per serving:

Carbohydrates – 2 g

Fat – 20 g

Protein – 46 g

Calories – 390

Ingredients:

- (6-ounce) boneless, skinless chicken breasts
- ½ cup commercially prepared pesto
- 2 ounces shredded part-skim mozzarella cheese (½ cup)
- Salt and freshly ground black pepper

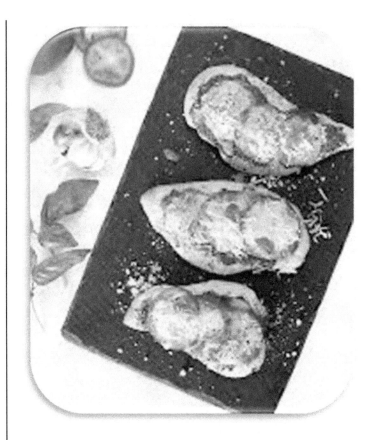

Instructions:

1. Heat oven to 375°F.
2. Season chicken with salt and pepper. Spread ¼ cup of the pesto in a 9-by-13-inch baking dish. Lay chicken breasts over pesto in an even layer and spread with remaining pesto.
3. Cover baking dish with foil and bake for 20 to 25 minutes. Uncover and top with cheese. Bake for 5 more minutes. Serve hot.

Baked Barbecue Chicken (Phase I)

Prep time: 10 minutes

Cooking time: 25 minutes

Servings: 4

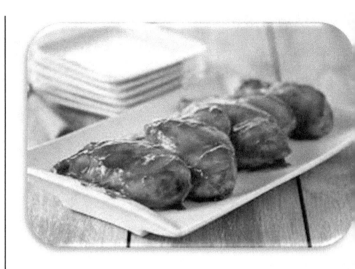

Nutrients per serving:

Carbohydrates – 2 g

Fat – 3.5 g

Protein – 40 g

Calories – 200

Ingredients:

- 4 (6-ounce) boneless, skinless chicken breasts
- 1 tsp extra-virgin olive oil
- ½ cup barbecue sauce
- Salt and freshly ground black pepper

Instructions:

1. Heat oven to 350°F.
2. Season chicken on both sides with salt and pepper.
3. In a skillet, heat olive. Add chicken and cook until browned, 2 minutes per side.
4. Place chicken, in a single layer, in an ovenproof baking dish and spoon sauce evenly over the top. Bake for 18 to 20 minutes.

The South Beach Diet

Ultimate Guide for Beginners with Healthy Recipes and Kick-Start Meal Plans

Emma Green

Phase I Meal Plan

Day 1

Breakfast	Chicken Salad in Cucumber Cups *(recipe on p. 91)* Fresh tomato juice with salt and pepper
Snack	Celery and cucumber sticks with hummus *(recipe on p. 97)*
Lunch	Grilled chicken breast with Indian spices
Snack	Roasted nuts (15 almonds/30 pistachios)
Dinner	Home-style dal *(recipe on p.104)* 1 stick mozzarella

Day 2

Breakfast	Hard-boiled eggs with boiled ham Decaffeinated tea or coffee
Snack	Turkey roll-ups *(recipe on p. 123)*
Lunch	Cauliflower soup Indian style *(recipe on p. 101)*
Snack	Roasted nuts (15 almonds/30 pistachios)
Dinner	2 fillets pecan-crusted cod with spinach *(recipe on p. 111)*

Day 3

Breakfast	1 slice quiche with spinach, mushrooms and bell peppers Fresh tomato juice with salt and pepper
Snack	Avocado guacamole *(recipe on p.98)*
Lunch	Pesto chicken breast *(recipe on p. 124)*
Snack	Roasted nuts (15 almonds/30 pistachios)
Dinner	Bok choy shrimp with stir-fried yellow squash *(recipe on p.115)*

Day 4

Breakfast	Omelet with chopped mushrooms 8 oz fat free milk
Snack	Roasted nuts (15 almonds/30 pistachios)
Lunch	Chicken kale soup *(recipe on p. 102)*
Snack	Cherry tomato salad *(recipe on p. 84)*
Dinner	Ground turkey salad *(recipe on p. 85)*

Day 5

Breakfast	1 slice Quiche with spinach, mushrooms and bell peppers *(recipe on p. 92)*. Fresh tomato juice with salt and pepper
Snack	Roasted nuts (15 almonds/30 pistachios)
Lunch	Spinach soup *(recipe on p. 103)* Cabbage stir-fry with Indian spices
Snack	Celery sticks with Cilantro Dip *(recipe on p. 100)*
Dinner	Baked chicken Cordon Bleu *(recipe on p. 125)*

Phase II Meal Plan

Day 1

Breakfast	1 slice cheddar broccoli quiche (recipe on p. 94)
Snack	1 container strawberries
Lunch	Tuna salad (recipe on p. 80)
Snack	Turkey deli meat with cucumber slices
Dinner	Ground turkey lettuce wraps (recipe on p. 130)

Day 2

Breakfast	1 slice Parmesan kale quiche *(recipe on p. 96)*
Snack	Greek yogurt with blueberries
Lunch	Split pea soup with Italian sausage *(recipe on p. 106)*
Snack	Celery sticks with cilantro dip *(recipe on p. 100)*
Dinner	Balsamic salmon *(recipe on p.112)*

Day 3

Breakfast	Fresh pineapple with cottage cheese
Snack	Greek yogurt
Lunch	Chinese hot and sour soup *(recipe on p. 109)*
Snack	Celery sticks with white cilantro dip *(recipe on p.100)*
Dinner	Asian marinade kebabs *(recipe on p. 131)*

Day 4

Breakfast	1 slice feta spinach quiche *(recipe on p. 95)*
Snack	1 banana
Lunch	Egg soup *(recipe on p. 108)*
Snack	Salmon cucumber bites *(recipe on p. 121)*
Dinner	Spinach stuffed chicken *(recipe on p. 134)*

Day 5

Breakfast	Fresh strawberries with cottage cheese
Snack	1 cup soy milk
Lunch	Gazpacho *(recipe on p. 105)*
Snack	Cherry tomato salad *(recipe on p. 84)*
Dinner	Greek style chicken *(recipe on p. 127)*

Salads

Tuna salad (Phase I)

Prep time: 10 minutes

Cooking time: none

Servings: 3

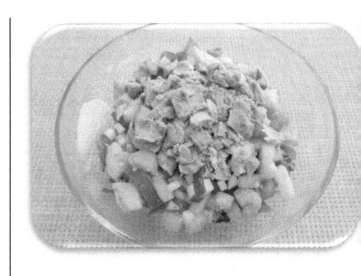

Nutrients per serving:

Carbohydrates – 4.8 g

Protein – 14.3 g

Total sugars – 1.1 g

Calories – 212

Ingredients:

- 1 can tuna (6 oz)
- ⅓ cup fresh cucumber, chopped
- ⅓ cup fresh tomato, chopped
- ⅓ cup avocado, chopped
- ⅓ cup celery, chopped
- 2 garlic cloves, minced
- 4 tsp olive oil
- 2 tbsp lime juice
- Pinch of black pepper

Instructions:

1. Prepare the dressing by combining olive oil, lime juice, minced garlic and black pepper.
2. Mix the salad ingredients in a salad bowl and drizzle with the dressing.

Roasted Portobello Salad (Phase I)

Prep time: 10 minutes

Cooking time: none

Servings: 4

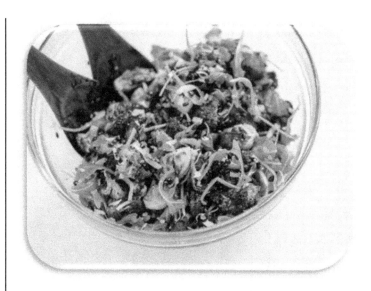

Nutrients per serving:

Carbohydrates – 22.3 g

Protein – 14.9 g

Total sugars – 2.1 g

Calories – 501

Ingredients:

- 1½ lb Portobello mushrooms, stems trimmed
- 3 heads Belgian endive, sliced
- 1 small red onion, sliced
- 4 oz blue cheese
- 8 oz mixed salad greens

Dressing:

- 3 tbsp red wine vinegar
- 1 tbsp Dijon mustard
- ⅔ cup olive oil
- Salt and pepper to taste

Instructions:

1. Preheat the oven to 450°F.
2. Prepare the dressing by whisking together vinegar, mustard, salt and pepper. Slowly add olive oil while whisking.
3. Cut the mushrooms and arrange them on a baking sheet, stem-side up. Coat the mushrooms with some dressing and bake for 15 minutes.
4. In a salad bowl toss the salad greens with onion, endive and cheese. Sprinkle with the dressing.
5. Add mushrooms to the salad bowl.

Shredded chicken salad (Phase I)

Prep time: 5 minutes

Cooking time: 10 minutes

Servings: 6

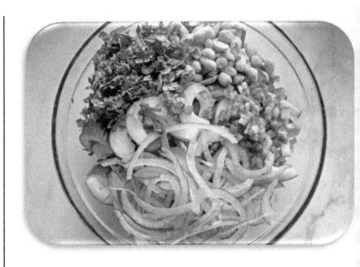

Nutrients per serving:

Carbohydrates – 9 g

Protein – 11.6 g

Total sugars – 4.2 g

Calories – 117

Ingredients:

- 2 chicken breasts, boneless, skinless
- 1 head iceberg lettuce, cut into strips
- 2 bell peppers, cut into strips
- 1 fresh cucumber, quartered, sliced
- 3 scallions, sliced
- 2 tbsp chopped peanuts
- 1 tbsp peanut vinaigrette
- Salt to taste
- 1 cup water

Instructions:

1. In a skillet simmer one cup of salted water.
2. Add the chicken breasts, cover and cook on low for 5 minutes. Remove the cover. Then remove the chicken from the skillet and shred with a fork.
3. In a salad bowl mix the vegetables with the cooled chicken, season with salt and sprinkle with peanut vinaigrette and chopped peanuts.

Broccoli Salad (Phase I)

Prep time: 10 minutes

Cooking time: none

Servings: 6

Nutrients per serving:

Carbohydrates – 17.3 g

Protein – 11 g

Total sugars – 10 g

Calories – 220

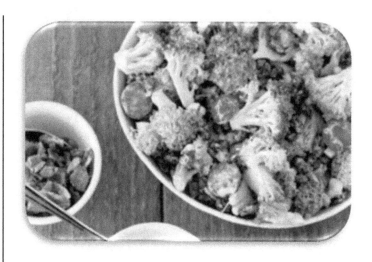

Ingredients:

- 1 medium head broccoli, raw, florets only
- ½ cup red onion, chopped
- 12 oz turkey bacon, chopped, fried until crisp
- ½ cup cherry tomatoes, halved
- ¼ cup sunflower kernels
- ¾ cup raisins
- ¾ cup mayonnaise
- 2 tbsp white vinegar

Instructions:

1. In a salad bowl combine the broccoli, tomatoes and onion.
2. Mix mayo with vinegar and sprinkle over the broccoli.
3. Add the sunflower kernels, raisins and bacon and toss well.

Cherry Tomato Salad (Phase I)

Prep time: 10 minutes

Cooking time: none

Servings: 6

Nutrients per serving:

Carbohydrates – 10.7 g

Protein – 2.4 g

Total sugars – 3.6 g

Calories – 259

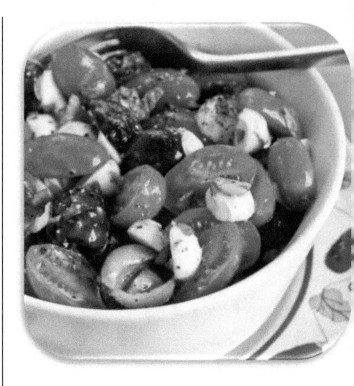

Ingredients:

- 40 cherry tomatoes, halved
- 1 cup mozzarella balls, halved
- 1 cup green olives, sliced
- 1 can (6 oz) black olives, sliced
- 2 green onions, chopped
- 3 oz roasted pine nuts

Dressing:

- ½ cup olive oil
- 2 tbsp red wine vinegar
- 1 tsp dried oregano
- Salt and pepper to taste

Instructions:

1. In a salad bowl, combine the tomatoes, olives and onions.
2. Prepare the dressing by combining olive oil with red wine vinegar, dried oregano, salt and pepper.
3. Sprinkle with the dressing and add the nuts.
4. Let marinate in the fridge for 1 hour.

Ground turkey salad (Phase I)

Prep time: 10 minutes

Cooking time: 35 minutes

Servings: 6

Nutrients per serving:

Carbohydrates – 9.1 g

Protein – 17.8 g

Total sugars – 2.5 g

Calories – 176

Ingredients:

- 1 lb lean ground turkey
- ½ inch ginger, minced
- 2 garlic cloves, minced
- 1 onion, chopped
- 1 tbsp olive oil
- 1 bag lettuce leaves (for serving)
- ¼ cup fresh cilantro, chopped
- 2 tsp coriander powder
- 1 tsp red chili powder
- 1 tsp turmeric powder
- Salt to taste
- 4 cups water

Dressing:

- 2 tbsp fat free yogurt
- 1 tbsp sour cream, non-fat
- 1 tbsp low fat mayonnaise
- 1 lemon, juiced
- 1 tsp red chili flakes
- Salt and pepper to taste

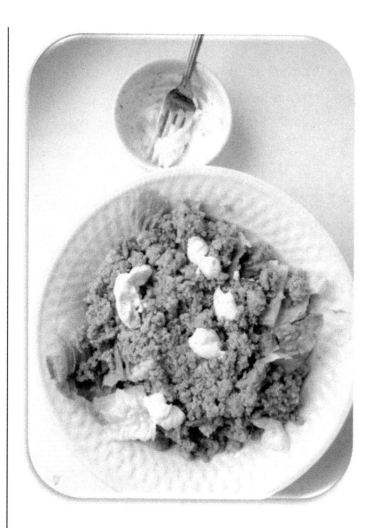

Instructions:

1. In a skillet sauté the garlic and ginger in olive oil for 1 minute. Add onion and season with salt. Cook for 10 minutes over medium heat.
2. Add the ground turkey and sauté for 3 more minutes. Add the spices (turmeric, red chili powder and coriander powder).
3. Add 4 cups water and cook for 30 minutes, covered.
4. Prepare the dressing by combining yogurt, sour cream, mayo, lemon juice, chili flakes, salt and pepper.
5. To serve arrange the salad leaves on serving plates and place the cooked ground turkey on them. Top with dressing.

Asian Cucumber Salad (Phase I)

Prep time: 10 minutes

Cooking time: none

Servings: 6

Nutrients per serving:

Carbohydrates – 5.7 g

Protein – 1 g

Total sugars – 3.1 g

Calories – 52

Ingredients:

- 1 lb cucumbers, sliced
- 2 scallions, sliced
- 2 tbsp sliced pickled ginger, chopped
- ¼ cup cilantro
- ½ red jalapeño, chopped
- 3 tbsp rice wine vinegar
- 1 tbsp sesame oil
- 1 tbsp sesame seeds

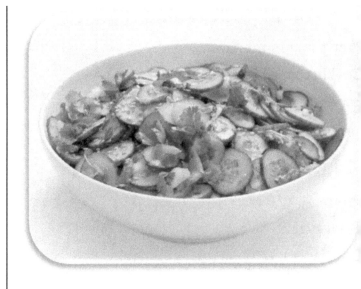

Instructions:

1. In a salad bowl combine all ingredients and toss together.

Cauliflower Tofu Salad (Phase I)

Prep time: 10 minutes

Cooking time: 15 minutes

Servings: 4

Nutrients per serving:

Carbohydrates – 34.1 g

Protein – 11.1 g

Total sugars – 11.5 g

Calories – 328

Ingredients:

- 2 cups cauliflower florets, blended
- 1 fresh cucumber, diced
- ½ cup green olives, diced
- ⅓ cup red onion, diced
- 2 tbsp toasted pine nuts
- 2 tbsp raisins
- ⅓ cup feta, crumbled
- ½ cup pomegranate seeds
- 2 lemons (juiced, zest grated)
- 8 oz tofu
- 2 tsp oregano
- 2 garlic cloves, minced
- ½ tsp red chili flakes
- 3 tbsp olive oil
- Salt and pepper to taste

Instructions:

1. Season the processed cauliflower with salt and transfer to a strainer to drain.
2. Prepare the marinade for tofu by

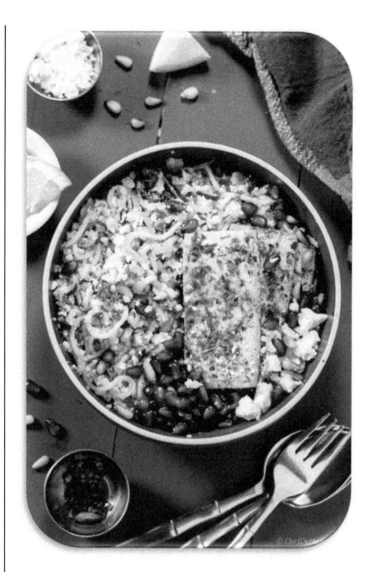

combining 2 tbsp lemon juice, 1.5 tbsp olive oil, minced garlic, chili flakes, oregano, salt and pepper. Coat tofu in the marinade and set aside.

3. Preheat the oven to 450°F.
4. Bake tofu on a baking sheet for 12 minutes.
5. In a salad bowl mix the remaining marinade with onions, cucumber, cauliflower, olives and raisins. Add in the remaining olive oil and grated lemon zest.
6. Top with tofu, pine nuts, feta and pomegranate seeds.

Scallop Caesar Salad (Phase I/II)

Prep time: 5 minutes

Cooking time: 2 minutes

Servings: 2

Nutrients per serving:

Carbohydrates – 14 g

Protein – 30.7 g

Total sugars – 2.2 g

Calories – 340

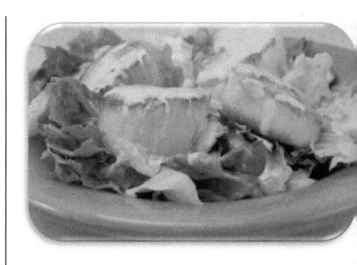

Ingredients:

- 8 sea scallops
- 4 cups romaine lettuce
- 2 tsp olive oil
- 3 tbsp Caesar Salad Dressing
- 1 tsp lemon juice
- Salt and pepper to taste

Instructions:

1. In a frying pan heat olive oil and cook the scallops in one layer no longer than 2 minutes per both sides. Season with salt and pepper to taste.
2. Arrange lettuce on plates and place scallops on top.
3. Pour over the Caesar dressing and lemon juice.

Chicken Avocado Salad (Phase I/II)

Prep time: 30 minutes

Cooking time: 15 minutes

Servings: 4

Nutrients per serving:

Carbohydrates – 10 g

Protein – 38 g

Total sugars – 11.5 g

Calories – 380

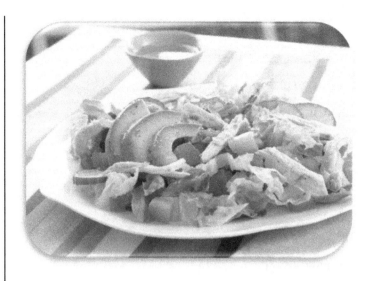

Ingredients:

- 1 lb chicken breast, cooked, shredded
- 1 avocado, pitted, peeled, sliced
- 2 tomatoes, diced
- 1 cucumber, peeled, sliced
- 1 head lettuce, chopped
- 3 tbsp olive oil
- 2 tbsp lime juice
- 1 tbsp cilantro, chopped
- Salt and pepper to taste

Instructions:

1. In a bowl whisk together oil, lime juice, cilantro, salt, and a pinch of pepper.
2. Combine lettuce, tomatoes, cucumber in a salad bowl and toss with half of the dressing.
3. Toss chicken with the remaining dressing and combine with vegetable mixture.
4. Top with avocado.

California Wraps (Phase I/II)

Prep time: 5 minutes

Cooking time: 15 minutes

Servings: 4

Nutrients per serving:

Carbohydrates – 4 g

Protein – 9 g

Total sugars – 0.5 g

Calories – 140

Ingredients:

- 4 slices turkey breast, cooked
- 4 slices ham, cooked
- 4 lettuce leaves
- 4 slices tomato
- 4 slices avocado
- 1 tsp lime juice
- A handful watercress leaves
- 4 tbsp Ranch dressing, sugar free

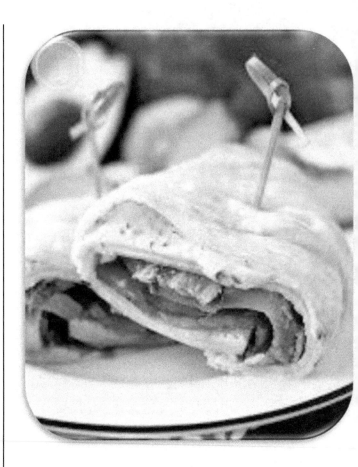

Instructions:

1. Top a lettuce leaf with turkey slice, ham slice and tomato.
2. In a bowl combine avocado and lime juice and place on top of tomatoes. Top with water cress and dressing.
3. Repeat with the remaining ingredients for
4. Topping each lettuce leaf with a turkey slice, ham slice, tomato and dressing.

Chicken Salad in Cucumber Cups
(Phase I)

Prep time: 5 minutes

Cooking time:15 minutes

Servings: 4

Nutrients per serving:

Carbohydrates – 4 g

Protein – 12 g

Total sugars – 0.5 g

Calories – 116

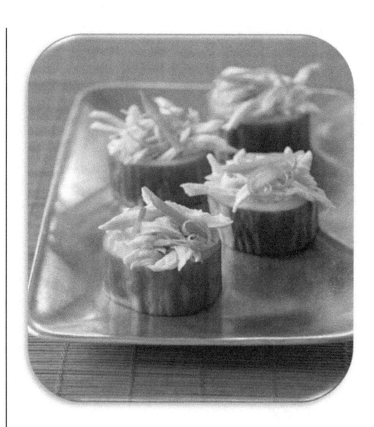

Ingredients:

- ½ chicken breast, skinless, boiled and shredded
- 2 long cucumbers, cut into 8 thick rounds each, scooped out (won't use in a recipe).
- 1 tsp ginger, minced
- 1 tsp lime zest, grated
- 4 tsp olive oil
- 1 tsp sesame oil
- 1 tsp lime juice
- Salt and pepper to taste

Instructions:

1. In a bowl combine lime zest, juice, olive and sesame oils, ginger, season with salt.
2. Toss the chicken with the dressing and fill the cucumber cups with the salad.

Quiches & Dips

Quiche with spinach, mushrooms and bell peppers (Phase I/II)

Prep time: 10 minutes

Cooking time: 1 hour

Servings: 6-8

Nutrients per serving:

Carbohydrates – 7.5 g

Protein – 16 g

Total sugars – 3.4 g

Calories – 138

Ingredients:

- 8 eggs
- ¼ cup milk, fat free
- 1 cup cottage cheese, low fat
- 2 cups any low fat cheese, grated
- 1 garlic, minced
- 2 cups spinach
- 3 cups mushrooms to your liking, diced
- 1 bell pepper, diced
- 1 cup red onions, diced
- 1 tsp red chili powder
- 1 tsp garam masala
- 1 tbsp olive oil
- Salt and pepper to taste

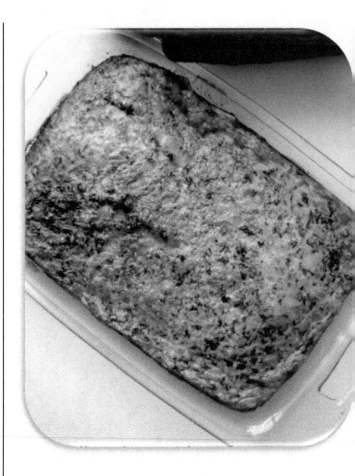

Instructions:

1. Beat the eggs with milk, add the cottage cheese and stir.
2. In a skillet sauté the garlic in the olive oil for about 30 seconds. Add the onions. Season with chili powder and garam masala.
3. Add the bell peppers, mushrooms and cook for 5 minutes. Add the spinach and sauté until wilted.
4. Preheat the oven to 375°F.
5. Spray a baking pan with some oil. Layer the sautéed vegetables, then the cheese. Pour the egg mixture over the pan making sure the liquid has evenly coated the vegetables.
6. Bake for 45 minutes.

Quiche Lorraine (Phase II)

Prep time: 10 minutes

Cooking time: 40 minutes

Servings: 6-8

Nutrients per serving:

Carbohydrates – 5.7 g

Protein – 25.6 g

Total sugars – 2 g

Calories – 372

Ingredients:

- 8 eggs
- 1 cup half and half
- ¼ cup bell pepper, diced, roasted
- 12 oz Swiss cheese, shredded
- 12 oz turkey bacon, crumbled
- 1 tsp parsley flakes
- ¼ tsp ground nutmeg
- Salt and pepper to taste

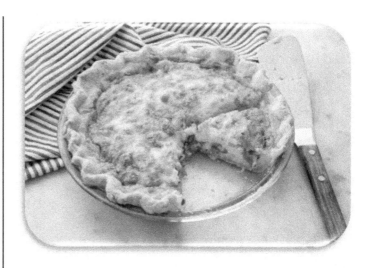

Instructions:

1. Preheat the oven to 350°F.
2. In a bowl mix eggs, half peppers and spices. Add the cheese and crumbled bacon.
3. Grease a baking pan and pour in the mixture. Bake for 40 minutes.

Cheddar Broccoli Quiche (Phase I)

Prep time: 10 minutes

Cooking time: 50 minutes

Servings: 6

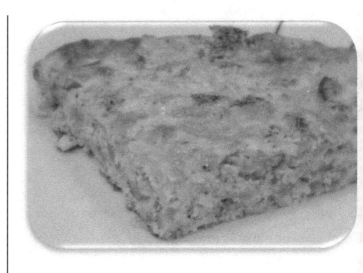

Nutrients per serving:

Carbohydrates – 4.8 g

Protein – 15 g

Total sugars – 2 g

Calories – 128

Ingredients:

- 2 cups egg beaters
- ½ cup cottage cheese, low fat
- ½ cup Cheddar, low fat, shredded
- ¼ cup onion, chopped
- 10 oz broccoli, chopped
- 1 tsp olive oil
- Salt and pepper to taste

Instructions:

1. Preheat the oven to 350°F.
2. In a skillet sauté onions in olive oil for 5 minutes, stirring. Add the broccoli and mix well.
3. Arrange broccoli and onions in a sprayed baking dish.
4. Mix the remaining ingredients until well blended and pour over the broccoli.
5. Bake for 50 minutes.

Feta Spinach Quiche (Phase I)

Prep time: 10 minutes

Cooking time: 25 minutes

Servings: 6

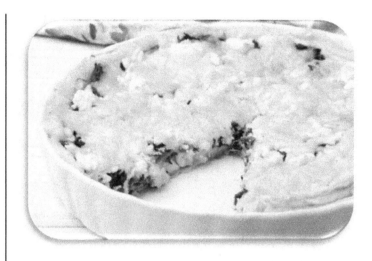

Nutrients per serving:

Carbohydrates – 13.7 g

Protein – 10.3 g

Total sugars – 2 g

Calories – 134

Ingredients:

- ½ cup egg beaters
- 2 eggs
- 1⅓ cups milk, low fat
- ½ cup feta cheese
- 1 onion, diced
- 8 oz baby spinach
- Salt and pepper to taste

Instructions:

1. In a skillet sauté onions in olive oil, stirring, for 5 minutes. Add the spinach and cook until wilted.
2. In a bowl whisk together eggs, egg beaters and milk. Add the spinach and onion mixture. Season with salt and pepper.
3. Preheat oven to 400°F.
4. Pour the quiche mixture into a greased baking dish. Top with feta.
5. Bake for 25 minutes.

Parmesan Kale Quiche (Phase I)

Prep time: 10 minutes

Cooking time: 40 minutes

Servings: 6-8

Nutrients per serving:

Carbohydrates – 5.4 g

Protein – 9.8 g

Total sugars – 2 g

Calories – 119

Ingredients:

- 2 eggs
- 1 bunch kale, ripped into small pieces
- ¼ cup sun-dried tomatoes, chopped
- 1 onion, chopped
- 1 cup cottage cheese
- ¾ cup Parmesan, grated
- 1 tbsp olive oil
- 1 tsp Dijon mustard
- 1 tbsp Italian seasoning

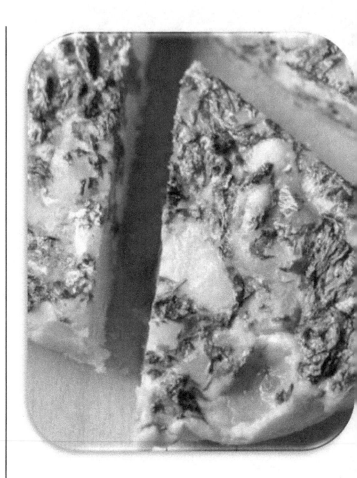

Instructions:

1. In a skillet sauté onions in olive oil, stirring, for 5 minutes. Add the kale and cook until wilted.
2. In a bowl whisk together eggs, cottage cheese, seasoning, mustard and Parmesan. Mix into the vegetables.
3. Preheat the oven to 375°F.
4. Pour the quiche mixture into a greased baking dish and bake for 40 minutes.

Plain Hummus (Phase I)

Prep time: overnight

Cooking time: 40 minutes

Servings: 4

Nutrients per serving:

Carbohydrates – 21.7 g

Protein – 10.1 g

Total sugars – 5.9 g

Calories – 340

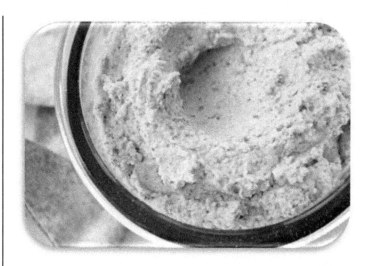

Ingredients:

- ½ lb chickpeas, soaked overnight
- 5 garlic cloves, minced
- 3 tbsp tahini paste
- 2 tbsp olive oil
- 2 tbsp lemon juice
- 1-2 tsp paprika powder
- 2 tsp mint, chopped
- Salt to taste
- 3 cups water

Instructions:

1. Prepare the soaked chickpeas by boiling in 3 cups of water until soft.
2. Grind the chickpeas together with garlic and olive oil.
3. Add the tahini paste and lemon juice. Season with salt and pepper.
4. Add the mint and mix well.
5. Store in the fridge and serve cold.

Avocado Guacamole (Phase I)

Prep time: 5 minutes

Cooking time: 3 minutes

Servings: 4

Nutrients per serving:

Carbohydrates – 4.2 g

Protein – 2 g

Total sugars – 1.7 g

Calories – 48

Ingredients:

- ⅓ avocado, peeled, mashed
- ⅓ cup cottage cheese, low fat
- 1 onion, chopped
- 1 garlic clove, minced
- ¼ cup cilantro, chopped
- 2 tbsp lemon juice
- ¼ tsp lemon zest, grated
- Salt and pepper to taste
- Celery sticks for serving

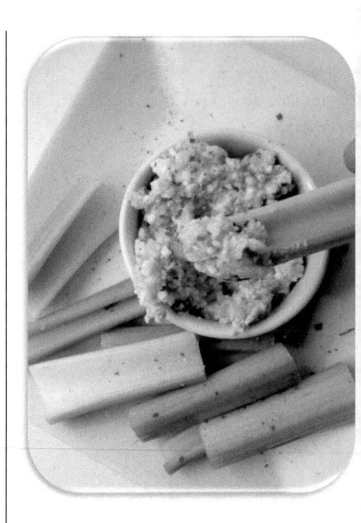

Instructions:

1. Mix all ingredients well and store in the fridge. Serve cool with celery sticks.

Note: can be enjoyed with whole wheat bread/crackers on Phase II

White bean dip (Phase I)

Prep time: 5 minutes

Cooking time:10 minutes

Servings: 4

Nutrients per serving:

Carbohydrates – 22.2 g

Protein – 7.5 g

Total sugars – 0.4 g

Calories – 179

Ingredients:

- 14 oz can white beans, rinsed
- 2 garlic cloves, chopped
- 10 black olives, pitted, chopped
- 2 tbsp parsley, chopped
- 2 tbsp olive oil
- 1½ tbsp lemon juice
- ¼ tsp dried oregano
- Pepper to taste

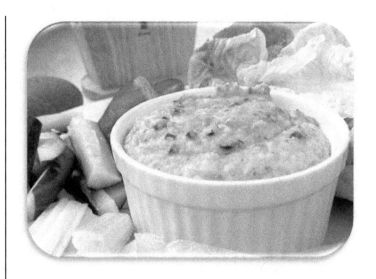

Instructions:

1. In a food processor purée the beans, garlic, parsley, oregano, lemon juice, olive oil and black pepper.
2. Transfer to a bowl, add olives and mix well.
3. Serve with celery or cucumber sticks.
4. Note: can be enjoyed with pita bread for Phase II

Cilantro Dip (Phase I/II)

Prep time: 5 minutes

Cooking time: 5 minutes

Servings: 8

Nutrients per serving:

Carbohydrates – 1 g

Protein – 1 g

Total sugars – 0.4 g

Calories – 100

Ingredients:

- 1 bunch cilantro, stems intact
- 1 garlic clove
- ⅓ cup walnuts, toasted
- 3 tbsp sour cream, reduced fat
- ¼ cup olive oil
- 2 tsp lemon juice
- Salt and pepper to taste

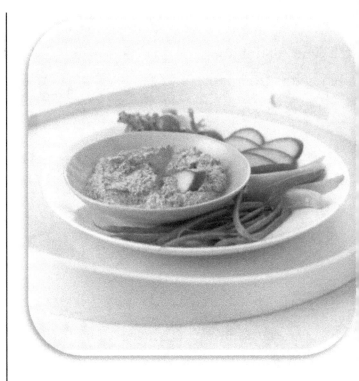

Instructions:

1. In a food processor purée the cilantro, garlic and walnuts.
2. Add oil, sour cream, lemon juice and season with salt and pepper. Pulse to combine.

Soups

Cauliflower Soup Indian Style (Phase I)

Prep time: 10 minutes

Cooking time: 40 minutes

Servings: 4

Nutrients per serving:

Carbohydrates – 18.5 g

Protein – 7.5 g

Total sugars – 5.8 g

Calories – 155

Ingredients:

- 1 head cauliflower, cut into florets
- 1 onion, chopped
- 1 garlic clove, minced
- ½ inch ginger, minced
- ½ cup fresh cilantro, chopped
- 1 cup sour cream, fat free
- 2 tsp coriander powder
- 1 tsp chili powder
- Pinch of garam masala
- 1 tbsp olive oil
- 3 cups chicken stock or water

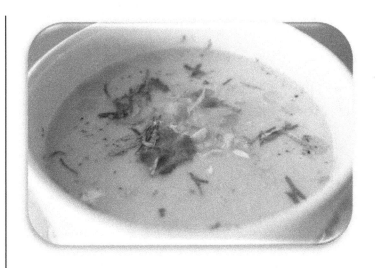

Instructions:

1. In a skillet sauté garlic and ginger in olive oil for about 40 seconds. add the onion and cook for 5 minutes. Season with coriander and chili powders.
2. Add the cauliflower and mix well.
3. Pour in the chicken stock or water and bring to a boil.
4. Cook for 20 minutes.
5. Transfer to a food processor and blend until smooth. Add sour cream and garam masala and pulse.
6. Serve with fresh cilantro.

Note: can be enjoyed with whole wheat crackers on Phase II.

Chicken Kale Soup (Phase I)

Prep time: 10 minutes

Cooking time: 40 minutes

Servings: 4

Nutrients per serving:

Carbohydrates – 18.5 g

Protein – 7.5 g

Total sugars – 5.8 g

Calories – 155

Ingredients:

- 3 cups chicken broth
- 1 cup chicken breast, skinless and boneless, cubed
- 1 bunch kale, chopped
- 1 cup red onion, diced
- 2 garlic cloves, minced
- 2 tsp red chili flakes
- 1 tsp thyme
- Salt and pepper to taste

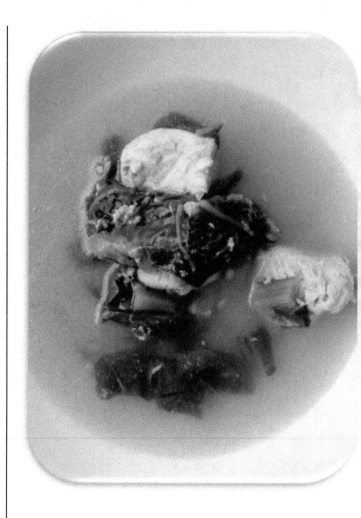

Instructions:

1. In a skillet sauté garlic in olive oil for about 40 seconds. Add the onion and cook for 5 minutes. Season with chili flakes.
2. Add the kale, chicken breast and sauté for 5 minutes.
3. Pour in the chicken stock and bring to a boil. Season with salt, pepper and thyme and cook for 30 minutes.

Spinach Soup (Phase I)

Prep time: 10 minutes

Cooking time: 40 minutes

Servings: 4

Nutrients per serving:

Carbohydrates – 3.2 g

Protein – 0.7 g

Total sugars – 2.2 g

Calories – 48

Ingredients:

- 1 cup spinach, chopped
- ¼ cup onion, chopped
- ¼ cup tomatoes, chopped
- 3 garlic cloves, minced
- 1 tbsp butter
- 2 tsp cumin seeds
- 1 tbsp lemon juice
- 3 cups water
- Salt and pepper to taste

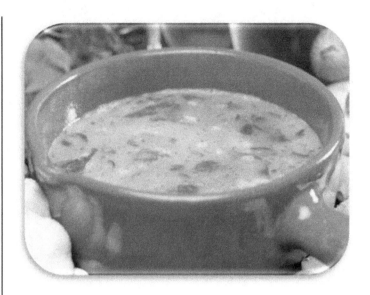

Instructions:

1. In a deep skillet sauté garlic in butter for about 40 seconds. Add the onion, tomatoes, spinach and cumin seeds and cook for 3 minutes. Season with salt and pepper.
2. Pour in the water and bring to a boil. Cook for 15 minutes.

Note: can be enjoyed with cooked rice on Phase II.

Home-style Dal (Phase I)

Prep time: 10 minutes

Cooking time: 40 minutes

Servings: 4

Nutrients per serving:

Carbohydrates – 12.3 g

Protein – 2.8 g

Total sugars – 1.3 g

Calories – 110

Ingredients:

- ½ cup garbanzo beans, rinsed
- 1 onion, chopped
- 8-10 fenugreek seeds
- ½ tsp turmeric powder
- Salt and ground coriander to taste
- 1½ tsp cow-milk ghee
- 1 tsp cumin seeds
- 5-6 curry leaves
- 2 green chilies, seeded, chopped
- 1½ cups water

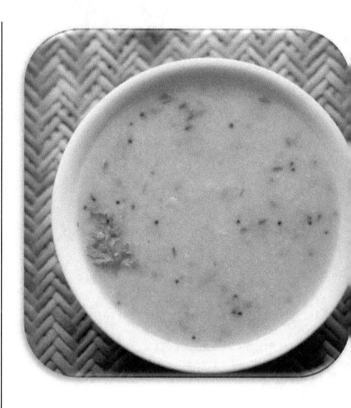

Instructions:

1. Add the rinsed beans to the pressure cooker, pour water. Add turmeric, fenugreek and onion and pressure cook on high for 10 min.
2. In a deep pan heat the ghee, add cumin seeds, curry leaves and chilies.
3. Add the cooked beans and season with salt and coriander. Simmer for 5 minutes. Add water in case you find the dal too thick.

Gazpacho (Phase I/II)

Prep time: 10 minutes

Cooking time: 15 minutes

Servings: 6

Nutrients per serving:

Carbohydrates – 12.6 g

Protein – 2.9 g

Total sugars – 5.5 g

Calories – 135

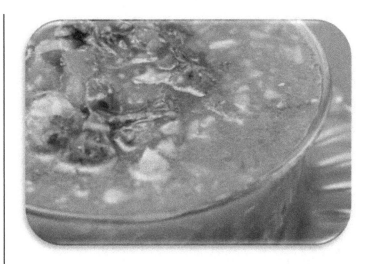

Ingredients:

- 3 red tomatoes, diced
- 3 yellow tomatoes, diced
- 1 cucumber, peeled, diced
- 1 onion, diced
- 2 celery stalks, diced
- 1 red sweet pepper, diced
- 1 tsp minced garlic
- ¼ cup red wine vinegar
- 3 tbsp basil, chopped
- 3 tbsp parsley, chopped
- ¼ cup olive oil
- 2 tbsp lemon juice
- 1 tsp Worcestershire sauce
- 2 cups tomato juice
- Salt and pepper to taste

Instructions:

1. In a food processor pulse the tomatoes, garlic and salt until desired consistency.
2. Put red wine vinegar and tomato mixture into a large pot.
3. In a food processor pulse cucumbers and onion. Add to the pot.
4. Repeat with the celery and red pepper. Add to the pot.
5. Add in basil, parsley, olive oil, lemon juice, Worcestershire sauce and tomato juice.
6. Season with pepper and check for consistency. If gazpacho is too thick for you, add more tomato juice.
7. Serve cool.

Split Pea Soup with Italian Sausage (Phase I/II)

Prep time: 10 minutes

Cooking time: 50 minutes

Servings: 6

Nutrients per serving:

Carbohydrates – 49.5 g

Protein – 35.5 g

Total sugars – 10.6 g

Calories – 477

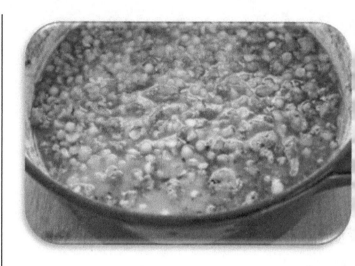

Ingredients:

- 2 cups yellow split peas
- 5 links turkey Italian sausage, cubed
- 1 onion, diced
- 1 cup celery, diced
- 1 green bell pepper, diced
- 1 tbsp minced garlic
- 2 tbsp olive oil
- 1 tsp Italian herb blend
- ½ tsp fennel seeds
- 6 cups chicken stock
- Salt and pepper to taste

Instructions:

1. In a large pot heat 1 tbsp olive oil and sauté onion, celery and green pepper for 3-4 min.
2. Add garlic, Italian herb blend and fennel seeds to the pot.
3. In a saucepan heat 1 tbsp olive oil and sauté the sausages, breaking them apart, until golden.
4. Add sausages to the pot of vegetables along with the split peas and chicken stock. Season with salt and pepper.
5. Bring to a boil and let simmer until the peas are soft.

Stuffed Peppers Soup (Phase I)

Prep time: 10 minutes

Cooking time: 50 minutes

Servings: 6

Nutrients per serving:

Carbohydrates – 28.1 g

Protein – 41.7 g

Total sugars – 6.3 g

Calories – 438

Ingredients:

- 2 green bell peppers, seeded, chopped into ½ inch cubes
- 5 links turkey Italian sausage
- 1 lb ground beef, lean
- 1 onion, chopped
- 2 cans (15 oz) crushed tomatoes
- 4 tsp olive oil
- 1 tbsp Italian herb blend
- 1 tbsp Worcestershire sauce
- ½ cup ketchup
- Salt and pepper to taste
- 7 cups beef stock
- Parmesan cheese for serving

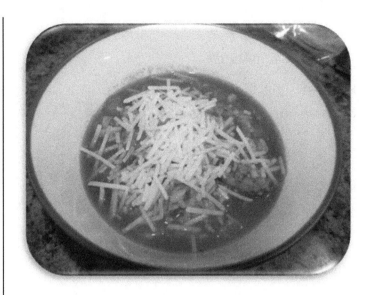

Instructions:

1. In a frying pan heat 2 tsp olive oil and sauté onion until golden. Season with Italian herb blend.
2. Transfer the onions into a large pot.
3. In the same frying pan sauté bell peppers for 3-4 min and add to the pot.
4. Add 2 more tsp olive oil to the frying pan and add the sausages and ground beef. Cook until browned breaking apart as it cooks.
5. Add beef and sausages to the pot.
6. Add the tomatoes, beef broth, Worcestershire sauce, and ketchup and bring to a boil.
7. Let simmer for 40 minutes.
8. Serve hot with Parmesan if desired.

Egg Soup (Phase I)

Prep time: 10 minutes

Cooking time: 50 minutes

Servings: 6

Nutrients per serving:

Carbohydrates – 28.1 g

Protein – 41.7 g

Total sugars – 6.3 g

Calories – 438

Ingredients:

- 1 egg
- 1 egg white
- 4 tbsp green onion, chopped
- 2 cups chicken broth
- 2 tsp soy sauce
- Pepper to taste

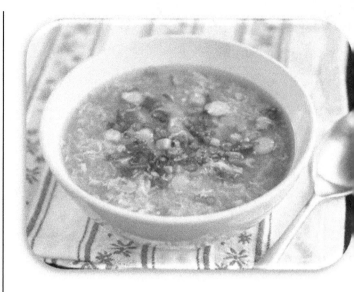

Instructions:

1. In a bowl beat a whole egg with the egg white.
2. Pour the chicken broth into a pot and bring to a boil.
3. Add green onions and remove from the heat.
4. Stir in the beaten egg gradually. Then add soy sauce and season with pepper.
5. Serve hot.

Chinese Hot and Sour Soup (Phase I)

Prep time: 10 minutes

Cooking time: 50 minutes

Servings: 5

Nutrients per serving:

Carbohydrates – 3.4 g

Protein – 13.4 g

Total sugars – 1.6 g

Calories – 90

Ingredients:

- 4 oz chicken breast, cooked, cut into strips
- ½ cup mushrooms, sliced
- 1 egg, beaten
- 1 tsp minced ginger
- ⅓ cup bamboo shoots, canned, cut into strips
- ¼ cup scallions, chopped
- ⅓ cup fresh snow pea pods
- ¼ cup rice vinegar
- ¼ cup soy sauce, low carb
- ½ tsp hot sauce
- 5 cups chicken broth
- Salt and pepper to taste

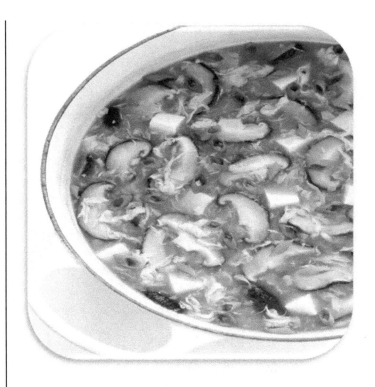

Instructions:

1. In a large pot combine chicken broth, mushrooms and ginger and bring to a boil.
2. Add chicken strips and let simmer for 10 minutes.
3. Add bamboo shoots and simmer for 5 minutes.
4. Add vinegar, soy sauce and hot sauce and bring to a boil again.
5. Add scallions and snow peas and cook for 1 minute. Take off the heat.
6. Slowly stir in the egg.
7. Season with pepper and top with more scallions, if desired.

Creamy Celery Cheddar Soup
(Phase I)

Prep time: 10 minutes

Cooking time: 50 minutes

Servings: 4

Nutrients per serving:

Carbohydrates – 14.3 g

Protein – 18 g

Total sugars – 5.7 g

Calories – 335

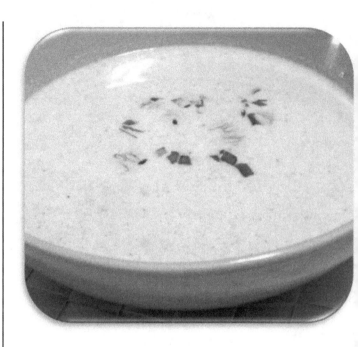

Ingredients:

- 3 tomatoes, chopped
- 1 celery stalk, chopped
- 2 green onions, chopped
- 1 tsp basil
- ¼ tsp onion powder
- 1 cup half & half
- 3 cups chicken stock
- 1½ cups Cheddar, shredded
- Salt and pepper to taste

Instructions:

1. In a food processor combine and purée 1 cup chicken stock, tomatoes, celery and green onions.
2. Pour 2 cups chicken stock into a soup pot and bring to a boil.
3. Add the processed vegetables and bring to a boil again.
4. Stir in half & half and season with basil, onion powder, salt and pepper.
5. Let simmer for 5 minutes, then add cheese and stir until melted.

Fish & Seafood

Pecan Crusted Cod (Phase I)

Prep time: 10 minutes

Cooking time: 20 minutes

Servings: 4

Nutrients per serving:

Carbohydrates – 2.2 g

Protein – 22.3 g

Total sugars – 0.6 g

Calories – 228

Ingredients:

- 4 cod fillets
- ¼ cup pecans, roasted
- 1 garlic clove
- 1 egg white, beaten
- 1 tsp red chili powder
- 1 tsp dried rosemary
- 2 tbsp olive oil
- Salt to taste

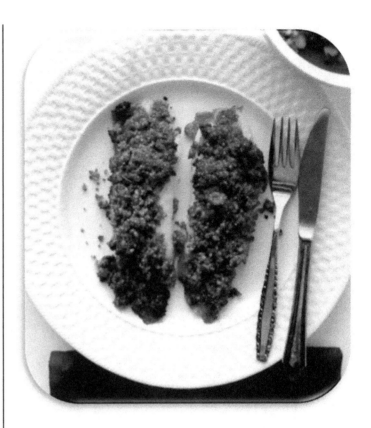

Instructions:

1. In a food processor finely chop the pecans, rosemary, garlic and chili powder.
2. Preheat the oven to 400°F.
3. Place the fish fillets on a baking sheet and season with salt. Brush with egg white and sprinkle with nut mixture.
4. Bake about 20 minutes.

Balsamic Salmon (Phase I/II)

Prep time: 10 minutes

Cooking time: 30 minutes

Servings: 2

Nutrients per serving:

Carbohydrates – 8.1 g

Protein – 43.5 g

Total sugars – 0.6 g

Calories – 306

Ingredients:

- 2 salmon fillets
- ½ cup balsamic vinegar
- ½ tsp lemon juice
- 1 tsp olive oil
- Salt and pepper to taste

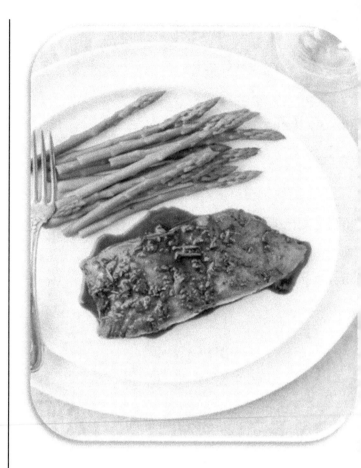

Instructions:

1. Preheat the oven to 450°F.
2. Season the fish fillets with salt and pepper, and place in a baking dish. Cover with foil. Bake for 15 minutes.
3. Prepare the balsamic glaze by stirring the vinegar over medium heat until reduced by about two-thirds. Add the lemon juice and olive oil.
4. Coat the salmon with glaze and serve.
5. Serve with asparagus for Phase I or with cooked rice for Phase II.

Cedar Plank Salmon (Phase I)

Prep time: 5 minutes

Cooking time: 20 minutes

Servings: 2

Nutrients per serving:

Carbohydrates – 10.6 g

Protein – 42.4 g

Total sugars – 9.3 g

Calories – 438

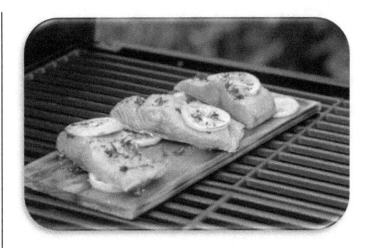

Ingredients:

- 2 salmon fillets
- 1 tsp cumin powder
- 1 tsp smoked paprika
- ½ tsp dried thyme
- ½ tsp garlic powder
- 1 tbsp olive oil
- Salt and pepper to taste

Instructions:

1. Prepare the grill by soaking cedar planks in water for at least 1 hour and preheating the grill.
2. In a bowl mix all dry ingredients and 1 tbsp olive oil. Combine to make a paste and rub it all over the salmon.
3. Place the fish on cedar planks and arrange on a grill over medium heat.
4. Cover and smoke for 20 minutes.

Tilapia Ceviche (Phase I)

Prep time: 3 hours

Cooking time: 10 minutes

Servings: 4

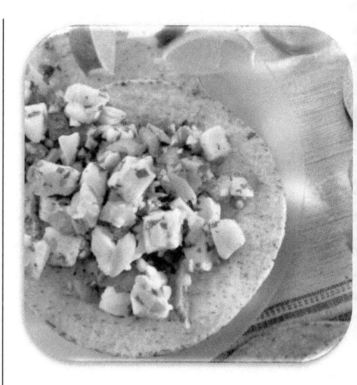

Nutrients per serving:

Carbohydrates – 9.9 g

Protein – 13 g

Total sugars – 3.4 g

Calories – 87

Ingredients:

- 2 tilapia fillets, diced
- 2 Roma tomatoes, diced
- 3 limes, juiced
- ½ onion, diced
- ½ tsp red chili garlic paste
- 2½ tbsp cilantro, chopped
- Salt and pepper to taste

Instructions:

1. Marinate the diced fish fillets in lime juice for 3 hours in the refrigerator.
2. Drain the liquid from the fish and set it aside. Mix the chili paste, tomatoes, onion and some of the lime juice, and then mix it with the fish. Season with salt and pepper.

Note: can be served with tortilla chips for Phase II.

Bok Choy Shrimp (Phase I)

Prep time: 5 minutes

Cooking time: 20 minutes

Servings: 4

Nutrients per serving:

Carbohydrates – 3.9 g

Protein – 10.1 g

Total sugars – 1.6 g

Calories – 95

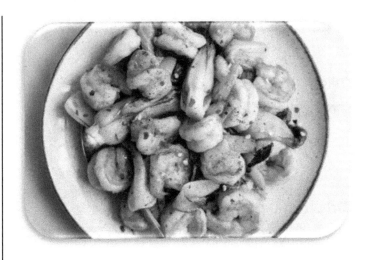

Ingredients:

- 20 shrimp, cleaned, deveined
- 3 bok choy bunches, chopped, use both stalks and leaves
- 1 onion, sliced
- 1 tbsp olive oil
- 1 tbsp soy sauce
- 2 garlic cloves, minced
- 2 tsp red chili flakes
- Salt and pepper to taste

Instructions:

1. In a skillet sauté garlic in olive oil for 30 seconds. Add onions and chili flakes and cook for 2-3 minutes more.
2. Add the shrimp and cook for 5 minutes.
3. After 5 minutes remove the shrimp and add the bok choy and soy sauce and cook for 5 minutes or until tender.
4. Season with salt and pepper and add shrimp back to the pan.
5. Stir and serve.

Chipotle Shrimp with Zucchini Noodles (Phase I)

Prep time: 15 minutes

Cooking time: 8 minutes

Servings: 4

Nutrients per serving:

Carbohydrates – 10.4 g

Protein – 43.6 g

Total sugars – 2.4 g

Calories – 316

Ingredients:

- 20 shrimp, cleaned, deveined
- 2 chipotle peppers
- 1 tbsp Adobo sauce
- 1 tbsp agave syrup
- 2 tbsp olive oil + 1 tsp for sautéing
- 2 garlic cloves
- ½ tsp cumin powder
- 1 tsp oregano
- 3 zucchini, spiralized
- Salt and pepper to taste

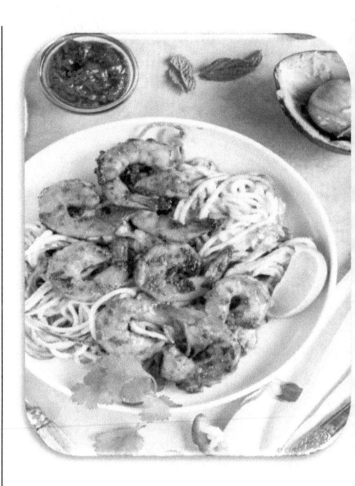

Instructions:

1. In a food processor blend chipotles, adobo, 1 tbsp olive oil, 1 tbsp agave syrup, 2 garlic cloves, cumin powder and oregano.
2. Coat shrimp in the chipotle sauce.
3. In a skillet sauté the zucchini in olive oil, season with salt and pepper.
4. Remove the cooked zucchini from the pan and add the marinated shrimp to the same pan. Cook for 2-3 minutes on each side.

Red Fish Stew (Phase I/II)

Prep time: 15 minutes

Cooking time: 30 minutes

Servings: 6

Nutrients per serving:

Carbohydrates – 7.1 g

Protein – 55.1 g

Total sugars – 4.4 g

Calories – 335

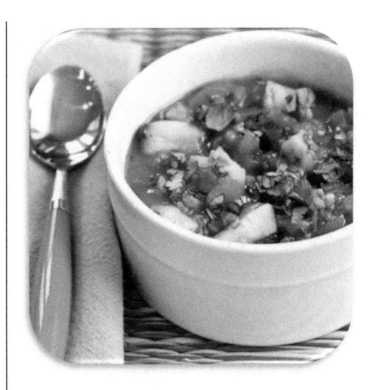

Ingredients:

- 8 (10 oz) cod, tilapia or halibut fillets, cut into 1 inch cubes
- ½ cup red onion, chopped
- 12 oz red bell peppers, chopped
- 1 can (14.5 oz) tomatoes, diced, with juice
- 1 tsp minced garlic
- 1 tbsp olive oil
- ¼ tsp red pepper flakes
- ¼ cup fresh cilantro, chopped
- ½ tsp lemon zest, grated
- 2 tsp lemon juice
- Salt and pepper to taste

Instructions:

1. In a skillet sauté onion in olive oil for 3-4 minutes. Add bell peppers, tomatoes with juice, garlic and red pepper flakes. Add some water if more liquid is required.
2. Let simmer for 10 minutes.
3. Add lemon juice and zest and ¼ cup cilantro.
4. Add fish and stir to combine.
5. Season with salt and pepper and let simmer for 10 minutes.
6. Serve with fresh cilantro.
7. Note: can be enjoyed with cooked rice for Phase II.

Almond and Parmesan Baked Fish (Phase I/II)

Prep time: 15 minutes

Cooking time: 30 minutes

Servings: 4

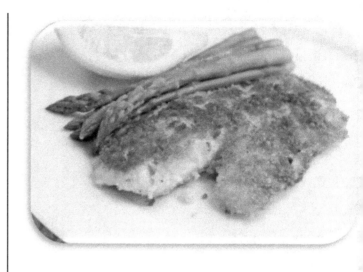

Nutrients per serving:

Carbohydrates – 1 g

Protein – 18.8 g

Total sugars – 0.2 g

Calories – 189

Ingredients:

- 4 white fish fillets, ½ inch thick
- ⅓ cup almond meal
- ¼ cup butter, melted
- 2 tbsp Parmesan, grated
- ½ tsp garlic powder
- Salt and pepper to taste
- ½ tsp fish rub

Instructions:

1. Preheat oven to 425°F.
2. In a bowl mix the almond meal, Parmesan, garlic powder, salt, pepper and fish rub.
3. Coat the fillets with butter all over; then dip into the almond meal mixture.
4. Bake for 20-30 minutes.

Fish & Cabbage Bowls (Phase I/II)

Prep time: 15 minutes

Cooking time: 30 minutes

Servings: 4

Nutrients per serving:

Carbohydrates – 13 g

Protein – 15.5 g

Total sugars – 7.6 g

Calories – 178

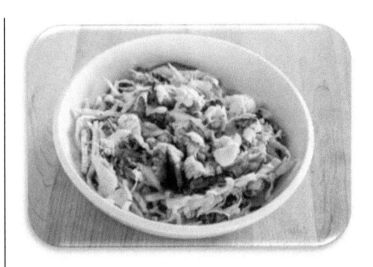

Ingredients:

- 3 white fish fillets
- 1 head green cabbage, sliced thin
- ½ head red cabbage, sliced thin
- ½ cup green onions, sliced
- 4 tsp olive oil
- 2 tsp fish rub
- 1 tsp ground cumin
- ½ tsp chili powder
- ½ cup mix of mayonnaise and plain Greek yogurt
- 2 tbsp lime juice
- 2 tsp green Tabasco Sauce
- Salt and pepper to taste

Instructions:

1. Mix together fish rub, ground cumin, and chili powder.
2. Rub the fish fillets with olive oil and dip into fish rub mixture.
3. Prepare the dressing by mixing mayo, Greek yogurt, lime juice and green Tabasco Sauce. Season with salt and pepper.
4. Preheat a frying pan with 2 tsp olive oil and cook fish on both sides for 8-10 minutes total.
5. Mix half the green onions with the green and red cabbage and stir in some dressing to moisten the cabbage.
6. When the fish is done, shred it apart with a fork.
7. Arrange the cabbage mixture in a bowl and top with fish. Drizzle over some dressing.
8. Serve with the remaining green onions.

Shrimp Cocktail

Prep time: 5 minutes

Cooking time: 15 minutes

Servings: 6

Nutrients per serving:

Carbohydrates – 4.3 g

Protein – 13.7 g

Total sugars – 2.6 g

Calories – 85

Ingredients:

- 30 shrimp, boiled and peeled
- ½ cup low-sugar ketchup
- 2 tbsp tomato paste
- 3 tsp lemon juice
- 4 tsp cream-style horseradish

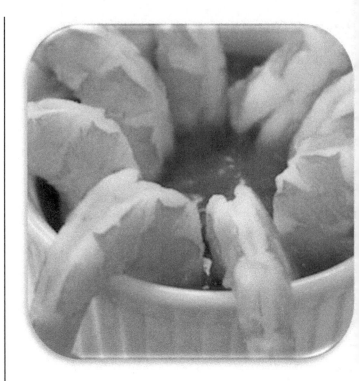

Instructions:

1. Stir together tomato paste and ketchup, add lemon juice and horseradish.
2. Serve shrimp with the cocktail sauce.

Salmon Cucumber Bites (Phase II)

Prep time: 5 minutes

Cooking time: none

Servings: 2

Nutrients per serving:

Carbohydrates – 4 g

Protein – 10 g

Total sugars – 2.6 g

Calories – 110

Ingredients:

- 3 oz pink salmon, canned
- 16 slices cucumber
- 1 tbsp celery, minced
- 1 tbsp onion, minced
- 1 tbsp mayonnaise
- ½ tsp yellow mustard
- 1 tsp fresh dill

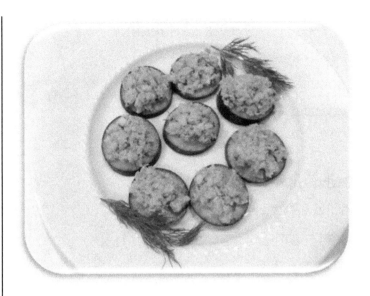

Instructions:

1. Combine all ingredients except the cucumbers and stir.
2. Spoon salmon mixture on each cucumber slice and serve.

Spicy Mussels

Prep time: 5 minutes

Cooking time: 15 minutes

Servings: 4

Nutrients per serving:

Carbohydrates – 16 g

Protein – 37 g

Total sugars – 2.6 g

Calories – 370

Ingredients:

- 4 lb mussels, beards removed
- 1 cup canned tomatoes, crushed
- 3 garlic cloves, minced
- 1 onion, chopped
- 2 tbsp olive oil
- 1 tsp basil, dried
- ¼ tsp red pepper flakes
- ½ cup water

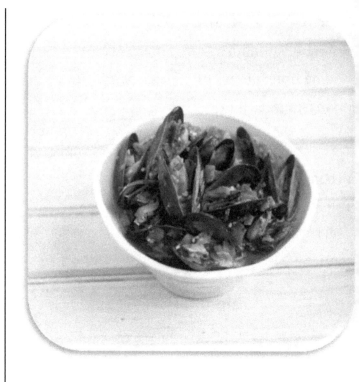

Instructions:

1. In a large skillet sauté onion, garlic and basil in olive oil for 3-4 min. Add pepper flakes.
2. Add water and bring to a boil, let simmer for 3 minutes.
3. Add tomatoes and mussels and cover. Cook for 8 minutes or until the mussels open.

Poultry

Turkey Roll-ups (Phase I)

Prep time: 5 minutes

Cooking time: 5 minutes

Servings: 4

Nutrients per serving:

Carbohydrates – 16.8 g

Protein – 9.1 g

Total sugars – 8.1 g

Calories – 126

Ingredients:

- 4 slices cooked turkey breast
- 4 lettuce leaves
- 4 scallions, diced
- 1 bell pepper, diced
- 4 small cucumbers, diced
- ¾ cup mayonnaise, low fat
- ¾ cup cilantro leaves, chopped
- 1 tbsp lime juice
- 1 tsp soy sauce
- 1 garlic clove, minced

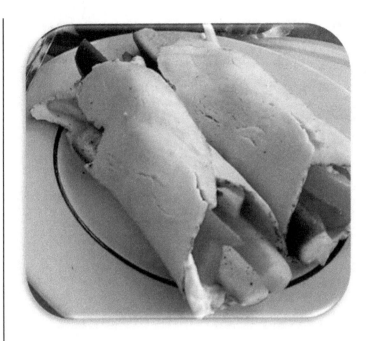

Instructions:

1. In a bowl mix mayo, cilantro, lime juice, soy sauce and garlic.
2. On each turkey slice, spread cilantro mayonnaise mixture, and then layer with lettuce, scallions, cucumber and peppers. Sprinkle with some more cilantro mayo mix and roll.

Pesto Chicken Breasts (Phase I/II)

Prep time: 5 minutes

Cooking time: 50 minutes

Servings: 4

Nutrients per serving:

Carbohydrates – 4.3 g

Protein – 30.3 g

Total sugars – 1.8 g

Calories – 287

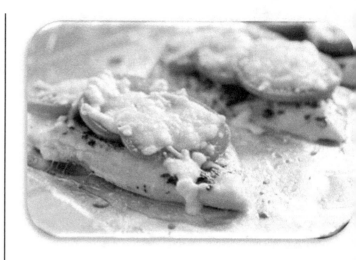

Ingredients:

- 4 chicken breasts, skinless
- 6 tbsp pesto
- 1 tomato, sliced
- 7 oz mozzarella cheese, grated
- 1 tbsp fresh parsley, chopped
- 1 tbsp fresh basil, chopped
- Salt and pepper to taste

Instructions:

1. Preheat the oven to 355°F.
2. Season the chicken breasts with pesto and salt and pepper.
3. Place into a baking dish and bake for 30 minutes.
4. Take the chicken out and sprinkle with mozzarella, tomatoes, basil and parsley, then mozzarella again.
5. Place the chicken back in oven for 20 more minutes.

Baked Chicken Cordon Bleu (Phase I)

Prep time: 15 minutes

Cooking time: 35 minutes

Servings: 4

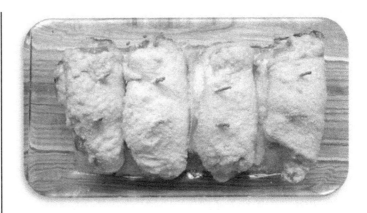

Nutrients per serving:

Carbohydrates – 1.7 g

Protein – 42.1 g

Total sugars – 1.1 g

Calories – 294

Ingredients:

- 4 chicken breasts, skinless, halved into ⅓ inch thick pieces
- 8 slices boiled ham
- 2 oz mozzarella, shredded
- 1 egg
- 1 tbsp margarine, melted
- ⅓ cup Parmesan, grated
- Salt and pepper to taste

Instructions:

1. Preheat the oven to 355°F.
2. In a baking dish place one slice ham on a chicken breast half and top with some mozzarella.
3. Roll up and pin with a toothpick.
4. Repeat the layering with the remaining slices.
5. Beat an egg and mix with melted margarine. Season with salt and pepper. Pour over chicken rolls.
6. Sprinkle with grated Parmesan.
7. Bake for 35 minutes.
8. Serve sliced.

Chicken Breasts with Goat Cheese Stuffing (Phase I)

Prep time: 15 minutes

Cooking time: 20 minutes

Servings: 2

Nutrients per serving:

Carbohydrates – 4.4 g

Protein – 47.9 g

Total sugars – 1.1 g

Calories – 354

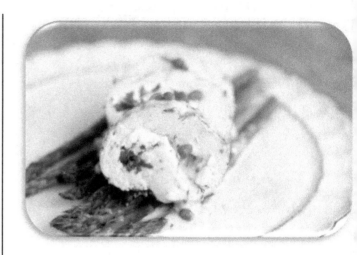

Ingredients:

- 2 chicken breasts, skinless, boneless
- 2 oz goat cheese, low fat
- 1 garlic clove, minced
- ½ bunch spinach
- 2 tsp olive oil
- Salt and pepper to taste

Instructions:

1. In a skillet sauté garlic in 1 tsp olive oil for 3 min.
2. Add spinach and cook for 3-4 minutes. Season with salt and pepper.
3. Cut out a pocket in each chicken breast and fill with spinach and cheese. Season breasts with salt and pepper.
4. Heat 1 tsp olive oil in the skillet and brown the chicken for 5 minutes.
5. Preheat the oven to 400°F. Transfer the chicken to a baking dish.
6. Bake for 10 minutes.

Greek style Chicken (Phase I/II)

Prep time: 2 hours

Cooking time: 20 minutes

Servings: 4

Nutrients per serving:

Carbohydrates – 2.2 g

Protein – 36.3 g

Total sugars – 0.4 g

Calories – 203

Ingredients:

- 1.5 lb chicken breasts, skinless
- 1 tbsp rosemary
- 1 tbsp oregano
- ½ tsp smoked paprika
- 4 tbsp lemon juice
- Salt and pepper to taste

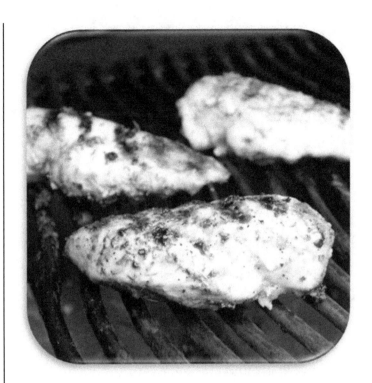

Instructions:

1. Season the chicken with spices and lemon juice and marinate for 2 hours.
2. Arrange the chicken on a grill and cook on each side until browned.

Ground Chicken and Chickpea Stew (Phase I/II)

Prep time: 5 minutes

Cooking time: 30 minutes

Servings: 6

Nutrients per serving:

Carbohydrates – 57.7 g

Protein – 30.8 g

Total sugars – 44.3 g

Calories – 379

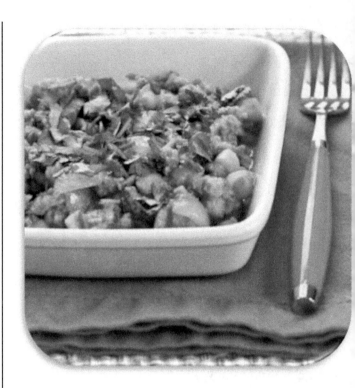

Ingredients:

- 1.5 lb ground chicken or turkey
- 1 onion, chopped
- 1 can (14.5 oz) tomatoes with juice, diced
- 1 can (16 oz) chickpeas
- 12 oz Greek yogurt, fat free
- 1 tbsp + 1 tsp olive oil
- 2 tbsp sweet curry powder
- Salt and pepper to taste

Instructions:

1. In a skillet heat 1 tbsp olive oil and add ground chicken or turkey breaking it apart as it cooks. Cook for about 8 minutes.
2. Add 1 tsp olive oil and chopped onion. Season with curry powder.
3. Add tomatoes with juice and chickpeas. Let simmer until the liquid evaporates.
4. Stir in yogurt and simmer for 3 more minutes.
5. Season with salt and pepper.

Saffron Chicken (Phase I/II)

Prep time: 5 minutes

Cooking time: 1 hour 10 minutes

Servings: 2

Nutrients per serving:

Carbohydrates – 9.8 g

Protein – 30.7 g

Total sugars – 4.1 g

Calories – 281

Ingredients:

- 2 chicken breasts, skinless, cut into large cubes
- 1 onion, cut into slices lengthwise
- 1 tbsp olive oil
- 1.5 tbsp lemon juice
- 1 tsp butter
- ¾ cup chicken stock
- Pinch saffron
- Salt and pepper to taste
- ¼ cup parsley, chopped

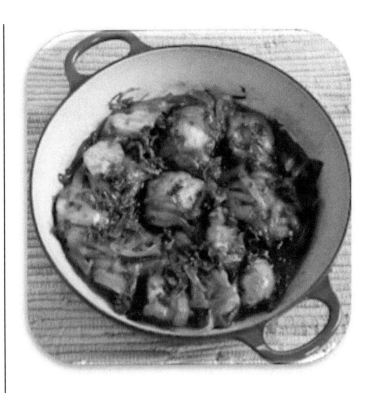

Instructions:

1. In a skillet brown the chicken in olive oil and butter.
2. Remove the chicken and add the onions to the pan; brown until golden over low heat.
3. Return chicken to the pan and cover with onions.
4. Add the stock and saffron, bring to a boil and let simmer for 45 minutes covered.
5. Add lemon juice, parsley and water if needed. Let simmer for 10 minutes.

Ground Turkey Lettuce Wraps (Phase I/II)

Prep time: 5 minutes

Cooking time: 1 hour 10 minutes

Servings: 6

Nutrients per serving:

Carbohydrates – 5.7 g

Protein – 28.4 g

Total sugars – 2.3 g

Calories – 174

Ingredients:

- 1.5 lb ground turkey
- 1 large head lettuce
- 3 tbsp onions, chopped
- 2 tbsp ginger root, grated
- 2 tbsp garlic, minced
- 1 tbsp olive oil
- 4 tbsp soy sauce
- 1 tbsp chili garlic sauce
- 1 cup cilantro, chopped

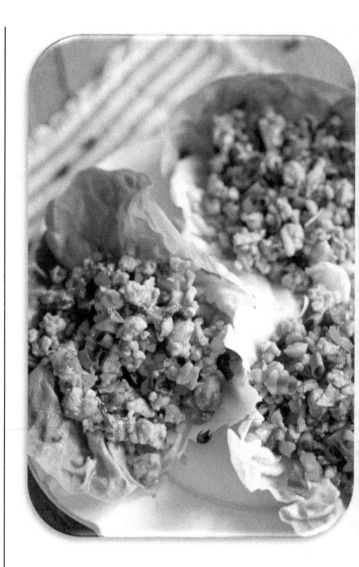

Instructions:

1. In a skillet sauté onions in olive oil for 2-3 minutes, add garlic and ginger root and sauté for 1 more minute.
2. Add ground turkey, breaking it apart as it cooks.
3. Add soy sauce and chili garlic sauce and cook until the turkey is brown.
4. Add chopped cilantro.
5. Take a lettuce leaf and fill it with turkey mixture and fold.

Asian Marinade Kebabs (Phase I/II)

Prep time: overnight

Cooking time: 20 minutes

Servings: 4

Nutrients per serving:

Carbohydrates – 4.7 g

Protein – 29.8 g

Total sugars – 1.7 g

Calories – 321

Ingredients:

- 4 chicken breasts, skinless, cut crosswise and cubed
- ¼ cup olive oil
- ¼ cup soy sauce
- 1 tbsp Asian sesame oil
- 1 tbsp garlic, minced
- 2 tsp ginger, grated
- 3 tbsp lime juice
- 1 tsp curry powder
- Salt and pepper to taste

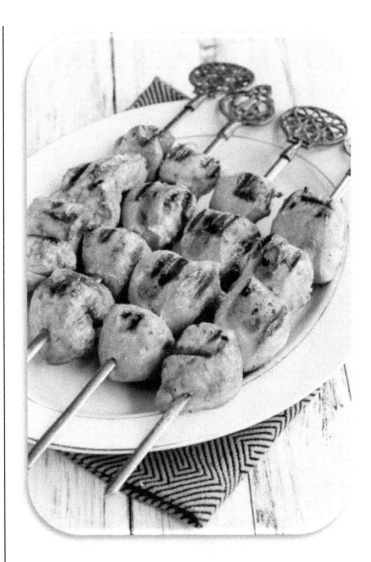

Instructions:

1. Make the marinade by mixing together olive oil, soy sauce, sesame oil, minced garlic, grated ginger, fresh lime juice, and curry powder.
2. Add chicken to a zip-lock bag and pour over the marinade. Marinate for 6-10 hours in the fridge.
3. Thread the chicken onto skewers and cook on a grill for 10 minutes.
4. Turn the skewers over and grill 5 minutes more.
5. Serve hot.

Tarragon Mustard Chicken (Phase I/II)

Prep time: overnight

Cooking time: 15 minutes

Servings: 4

Nutrients per serving:

Carbohydrates – 1.4 g

Protein – 29 g

Total sugars – 0.1 g

Calories – 317

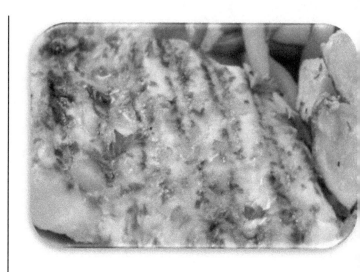

Ingredients:

- 4 chicken breasts, skinless, cut in half
- ⅓ cup olive oil
- 2 tbsp tarragon, chopped
- 2 tbsp Dijon mustard
- 1 tbsp fresh lemon juice
- 1 tsp minced garlic or garlic purée
- 1 tsp Spike Seasoning

Instructions:

1. In a food processor make the marinade by blending together tarragon, olive oil, mustard, lemon juice, garlic and Spike Seasoning.
2. Add chicken to a zip-lock bag and pour over the marinade. Marinate for 6-10 hours in the fridge.
3. Lay chicken breasts onto a preheated grill and cook, rotating, until chicken is browned and firm.
4. Serve hot.

Charmoula Sauce Chicken (Phase I/II)

Prep time: overnight

Cooking time: 15 minutes

Servings: 4

Nutrients per serving:

Carbohydrates – 2.1 g

Protein – 29.4 g

Total sugars – 0.7 g

Calories – 295

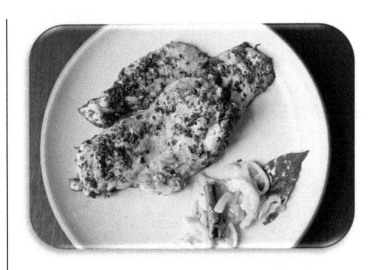

Ingredients:

- 4 chicken breasts, skinless, cut in half crosswise
- 2 garlic cloves, chopped
- ½ cup cilantro, chopped
- ¼ cup parsley, chopped
- 1 tbsp + 2 tsp lemon juice
- ½ tsp sweet paprika
- ½ tsp ground cumin
- 4 tbsp olive oil
- Salt and pepper to taste

Instructions:

1. Make the marinade by blending together chopped garlic, chopped cilantro, chopped parsley, lemon juice, sweet paprika, and ground cumin.
2. Add chicken to a zip-lock bag and pour over the marinade. Marinate for 6-10 hours in the fridge.
3. You can fry the chicken in a preheated pan or grill it on a preheated grill on all sides until golden.

Spinach Stuffed Chicken

Prep time: 5 minutes

Cooking time: 1 hour

Servings: 4

Nutrients per serving:

Carbohydrates – 9 g

Protein – 32 g

Total sugars – 0.7 g

Calories – 308

Ingredients:

- 4 chicken breasts, skinless
- 12 oz frozen spinach soufflé, cut into 4 equal parts
- 2 garlic cloves, sliced
- 2 tbsp olive oil
- 1 tsp Dijon mustard
- 2 tbsp lemon juice
- 1 cup chicken stock
- Salt and pepper to taste

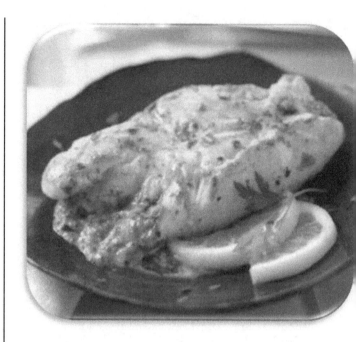

Instructions:

1. Top half of each chicken breast with spinach soufflé piece. Fold half of the chicken over the filling and pin with wooden picks.
2. In a skillet sauté garlic in olive oil until golden.
3. Remove the garlic and brown the chicken breasts for 7 minutes on each side.
4. Preheat the oven to 350°F.
5. Place the chicken onto a baking dish and bake for 40 minutes.
6. In a sauce pan heat the stock, lemon juice, mustard, salt and pepper. Add back the garlic. Bring to a boil and let simmer for 20 minutes.
7. Serve the chicken with the sauce, garnished with parsley.

CONCLUSION

Thank you for reading this book and having the patience to try the recipes.

I do hope that you have had as much enjoyment reading and experimenting with the meals as I have had writing the book.

If you would like to leave a comment, you can do so at the Order section->Digital orders, in your account.

Stay safe and healthy!

Recipe Index

Conversion Tables

VOLUME EQUIVALENTS (LIQUID)

US STANDARD	US STANDARD (OUNCES)	METRIC
2 tablespoons	1 fl. oz.	30 mL
¼ cup	2 fl. oz.	60 mL
½ cup	4 fl. oz.	120 mL
1 cup	8 fl. oz.	240mL
1½ cups	12 fl. oz.	355 mL
2 cups or 1 pint	16 fl. oz.	475 mL
4 cups or 1 quart	32 fl. oz.	1 L
1 gallon	128 fl. oz.	4 L

OVEN TEMPERATURES

FAHRENHEIT (°F)	CELSIUS (°C) APPROXIMATE
250 °F	120 °C
300 °F	150 °C
325 °F	165 °C
350 °F	180 °C
375 °F	190 °C
400 °F	200 °C
425 °F	220 °C
450 °F	230 °C

VOLUME EQUIVALENTS (LIQUID)

US STANDARD	METRIC (APPROXIMATE)
1/8 teaspoon	0.5 mL
¼ teaspoon	1 mL
½ teaspoon	2 mL
2/3 teaspoon	4 mL
1 teaspoon	5 mL
1 tablespoon	15 mL
¼ cup	59 mL
1/3 cup	79 mL
½ cup	118 mL
2/3 cup	156 mL
¾ cup	177 mL
1 cup	235 mL
2 cups or 1 pint	475 mL
3 cups	700 mL
4 cups or 1 quart	1 L
½ gallon	2 L
1 gallon	4 L

WEIGHT EQUIVALENTS

US STANDARD	METRIC (APPROXIMATE)
½ ounce	15 g
1 ounce	30 g
2 ounces	60 g
4 ounces	115 g
8 ounces	225 g
12 ounces	340 g
16 ounces or 1 pound	455 g

Other Books by Emma Green

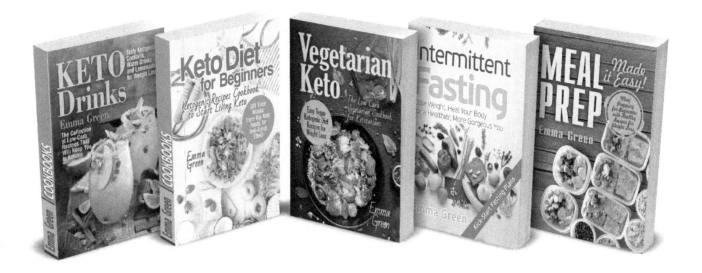

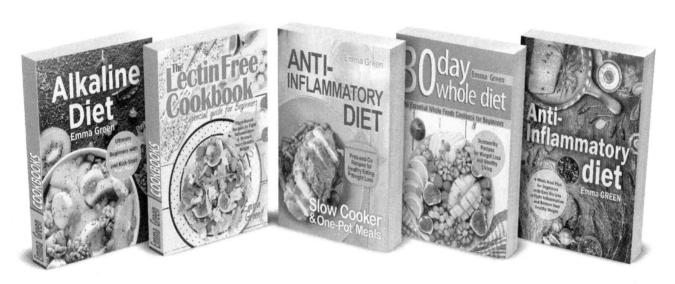

CPSIA information can be obtained
at www.ICGtesting.com
Printed in the USA
LVHW060741170220
647168LV00016B/170